3rd edition

# Healthy
## BEGINNINGS

Your handbook for pregnancy and birth

**Healthy Beginnings:** Your handbook for pregnancy and birth, 3rd edition

*Healthy Beginnings: Your handbook for pregnancy and birth is based on the SOGC Clinical Practice Guideline Healthy Beginnings: Guidelines for Care During Pregnancy and Childbirth, which was adapted for the public and written by* **Nan Schuurmans**, *MD, FRCSC, Edmonton, AB (SOGC President, 1996-97) and under the direction of* **André Lalonde**, *MD, FRCSC, Executive Vice-President, SOGC, Ottawa, ON.*

**Edited by:** Kelly Nolan and Michael Haymes, SOGC Ottawa
**Designed by:** Red Wagon Studio - Ottawa
**Illustrations:** Julie Dorion - Ottawa
**Copy editor:** Jacqueline Couture - Ottawa
**Consultants:** Past and present members of the SOGC
Kelly Anderson, MD, FRCPC, IBCLC, Pediatrician, Edmonton, AB
Louise Aubrey, RD, Health Canada Nutrition Unit, Ottawa, ON
Best Start: Ontario's Maternal, Newborn and Early Child
    Development Resource Centre
Shirley Gross, MD, CM, CCFP, The Edmonton Breastfeeding
    Clinic, Edmonton, AB
Montreal Diet Dispensary Dieticians, Montreal, QC
Jean-Marie Moutquin, MD, MSc, FRCSC, Laval, QC
Geeta Sukhrani, MD, FRCPC, Pediatrician, Edmonton, AB
Canadian Paediatric Society

**Acknowledgments:**
Irene Colliton, MD, Edmonton, AB
Brenda Dushinski, RN, Calgary, AB
Ahmed Ezzat, MD, FRCSC, Saskatoon, SK
Guy-Paul Gagné, MD, FRCSC, LaSalle, QC
Thomas Gleason, MD, FRCSC, Edmonton, AB
Catherine MacKinnon, MD, Brantford, ON
Gwen Peterek, RN, London, ON
Kathleen Wilson, RM, Ilderton, ON
Jennifer Wood for her invaluable help
    in preparation of the document.
Peel Public Health
Ontario Breastfeeding Committee
Sport C.A.R.E. Exercise and Pregnancy Education Program
Nutrition Resource Centre
Pregnets
Genetics Education Project
Perinatal Partnership Program of Eastern and
Southeastern Ontario
Centre for Addiction and Mental Health
Infant Mental Health Promotion
Ontario Society of Nutrition Professionals in Public Health
Motherisk
Diabetes Ontario
Canadian Foundation for the Study of Infant Deaths
Central South West Reproductive Health Working Group
Thunder Bay Midwives
Peterborough County-City Health Unit
Ottawa Public Health
Windsor-Essex County Health Unit
University of Ottawa
Registered Nurses Association of Ontario
The Hospital for Sick Children
Dr. Patricia Mousmanis, MD

**The Society of Obstetricians and Gynaecologists of Canada (SOGC)**
780 Echo Drive, Ottawa, ON K1S 5N8
Copyright © 1998, 2nd edition, 2000, 3rd edition, 2005

**Library and Archives Canada Cataloguing in Publication**
Schuurmans, Nan
   Healthy beginnings : your handbook for pregnancy and birth /
[written by Nan Schuurmans ; under the direction of André Lalonde ;
illustrations, Julie Dorion]. -- 3rd ed.

Includes index.
ISBN 1-897116-22-5

1. Pregnancy--Miscellanea. 2. Childbirth--Miscellanea. 3. Infants
   (Newborn)--Care--Miscellanea. I. Lalonde, André, 1943- II. Society of
   Obstetricians and Gynaecologists of Canada III. Title.

RG525.S34 2006   618.2   C2005-907545-7

# Important information

Name:

Phone:

**Health care provider:**        *Office phone:*

*Office nurse/secretary:*        *Answering service:*

**Pediatrician:**        *Phone:*

**Family physician:**        *Phone:*

**Hospital:**        *Phone:*

*Address:*

**Ambulance:**        *Phone:*

**Breastfeeding consultant:**        *Phone:*

**Public health nurse:**        *Phone:*

**Household help:**        *Phone:*

**Neighbour:**        *Phone:*

**Partner's phone during the day:**

**Expected delivery date:**

**Blood type:**

# Appointments with my health care providers

| Date | Day | Time |
|------|-----|------|
| First visit | | |
| | | |
| | | |
| | | |
| | | |
| | | |
| | | |
| | | |
| | | |
| | | |
| | | |
| | | |
| | | |
| | | |
| | | |
| | | |
| | | |
| | | |
| | | |
| | | |
| | | |
| | | |
| | | |

This handbook is written by the Society of Obstetricians and Gynaecologists of Canada to give women the information they need to make good choices in pregnancy. It is based on the Society's publication Healthy Beginnings: Guidelines for Care During Pregnancy and Childbirth, the guidelines Canadian doctors use in their practices to make decisions based on the most current research.

Being well informed about the ways your body prepares for birth and what your growing baby will need has been shown to make a big difference in how well your pregnancy progresses, and how healthy your newborn will be.

The advice and information in this handbook is "evidence based." This means that all the information in it is drawn from professional and credible research, rather than opinions or conjecture. The idea for this book came from international research showing that if pregnant women are aware of possible problems and how they can be prevented, mothers will have healthier pregnancies and more babies will be born full size, full term, and healthy.

## How to use this book

Use your Healthy Beginnings handbook to read about what is happening and what is about to happen. Write down any questions you still have and bring them to your next appointment. Use the journal spaces to take notes during your prenatal visits—especially if your partner is unable to accompany you.

Along with the standardized records your doctor's office keeps for you, the Healthy Beginnings handbook is an important part of your medical records. Record the changes in your body and your feelings for reference at the next office visit, or even months and years later, when your notes will remind you of this special time.

This book is not intended to replace the other good books, videos, audiotapes, or websites that your doctor or childbirth educator may recommend. No book can take the place of medical advice and prenatal care that are tailored to your particular needs.

Note to the reader:
Within this handbook, masculine and feminine pronouns have been used interchangeably for equal representation and health care provider may refer to doctors, midwives or nurses.

"One of the most gratifying parts of my everyday practice is helping women understand how their bodies work, and when something is wrong, explaining why and what we can do to remedy the problem.

Because we are often very busy, doctors and other health care providers cannot always explain everything that a woman may need to know to make the right decisions for her health.

I am hopeful that this book will give the information you need during your pregnancy and also help you in communicating with your doctor."

**Nan Schuurmans**, MD, FRCSC, FSOGC
Clinical Practice Obstetrics Committee

"This is a book for everyday use, to empower women to create a healthy beginning for their child, themselves, and their family."

**A.B. Lalonde**, MD, FRCSC, FSOGC, MSc,
Executive Vice-President, SOGC

## Table of Contents

# A healthy start to your family

## THE MENSTRUAL CYCLE

*The average menstrual cycle lasts 28 days. It may vary from 23–35 days. Almost every woman's cycle varies slightly from month to month.*

*Hormones produced by your body control the changes that occur throughout the cycle.*

*They cause an egg to mature in the ovary and control the timing of the release of the mature egg (ovulation). Ovulation occurs about 14 days before your next period.*

*Hormones also cause the lining of the uterus (endometrium) to become thick with a layer of specialized cells and tissue. If your partner's sperm has fertilized the egg, this layer of cells and tissues acts as a protective home for a fertilized egg to grow and develop into a baby. If fertilization does not happen, the body sheds this protective layer during your next period.*

*This chapter will help give you and your baby a head start if you are planning your family and hoping to become pregnant.*

*Most women understand how important it is to take good care of themselves and their unborn child once they are pregnant. You may not realize that what you eat and how you keep fit before you are pregnant will also make a difference. In this chapter, we'll look at how your body prepares itself for reproduction, and what you can do to improve your chances of having a normal pregnancy and a healthy baby.*

## It all begins with an egg

At a certain point during a woman's monthly menstrual cycle, an egg will be released from an ovary. This is called ovulation. The egg will begin to move down the fallopian tube toward the uterus. If a sperm meets with the egg and enters inside, fertilization takes place and the woman is pregnant. The fertilized egg begins to grow at once by dividing into two parts, then into four parts, then into eight parts, and so on.

It will continue to move down the fallopian tube as it grows, and within seven days the egg will bury itself into the thickened lining of the uterus, which is called the endometrium. This process of burrowing into the lining is called implantation. For the first eight weeks, the fertilized egg is called an embryo. After eight weeks, and until birth, the embryo is called a fetus.

Fertilized egg

Ovary

Uterus

Uterine cavity

Fallopian tube

Endometrium

Cervix

## How your body supports new life

Within your uterus, the growing baby has everything it needs to live. It is protected in a sac filled with amniotic fluid. Its supply line to the outside world is the placenta, an organ made up of blood vessels and tissue that is firmly attached to the lining of the mother's uterus.

The placenta is the system that connects the mother to the fetus. The placenta begins to develop as soon as implantation has taken place and continues to grow throughout the pregnancy. When blood passes from the mother to baby through the placenta, it allows for the exchange of beneficial oxygen, nutrients and protective antibodies. On the return trip, the blood picks up fetal waste products that will then be transported to the mother's bloodstream for removal by her organs.

The placenta also makes and secretes a number of hormones, including estrogen and progesterone. These hormones are responsible for many of the changes that occur in a woman's body during pregnancy. One of these important hormones, which only the placenta can produce, is called human chorionic gonadotrophin (HCG). A pregnancy test is considered positive if this hormone is found in a woman's urine or blood.

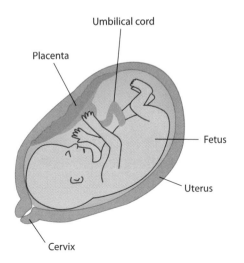

Umbilical cord

Placenta

Fetus

Uterus

Cervix

### EARLY SIGNS OF PREGNANCY

*Missed period.*

*Feeling unusually tired.*

*Tingling or tender breasts.*

*Need to urinate often.*

*Feeling bloated.*

*Nausea (morning sickness).*

*Any unusual bleeding (different from your normal period).*

*Any one of these signs, especially when combined with a missed period, could mean you are pregnant (even if you have been using a reliable form of birth control).*

### DID YOU KNOW?

*25% of women who have sexual intercourse without using birth control will get pregnant within one month*

*85% will become pregnant within one year*

*85% of babies arrive within a week before or a week after their due date*

1. *A rise in hormone levels causes ovulation to occur 14 days before next period.*

2. *Lining of uterus begins to thicken to prepare a safe home for a fertilized egg.*

3. *Mucus secreted from the cervix becomes more plentiful, clear, and slippery like raw egg white.*

4. *The egg is released from the ovary to begin its journey down the fallopian tube.*

5. *Body temperature rises for a few days just after ovulation.*

6. *Mild lower abdominal discomfort or bloating may be noted at ovulation.*

## Keep track of your monthly cycle

If you don't already keep a record of your menstrual cycle, this is a good time to start. Mark each day of your period on a calendar, and you will soon have a written record that will help you to know what is normal for you and to discover when you are most fertile—and therefore most likely to conceive. Once you become pregnant, your knowledge of your body's cycles will help your health care provider more accurately calculate the day your baby will be expected to be born (your due date). Your due date, and the date of your last menstrual period, is also used to measure how your baby is growing as the pregnancy progresses.

How easily you will become pregnant depends a great deal on your menstrual cycle. You are most fertile near the time of ovulation, and if you are hoping to become pregnant, you and your partner will want to have sexual intercourse around that time. But how can you tell when you are ovulating? The easiest way to tell when you will ovulate is to count back 14 days from the day when you predict your next period will start. Most women don't have to do anything different to get pregnant—for most, it happens naturally.

If you need to be more sure of the best days to try to get pregnant, you can watch for changes in your body that signal ovulation (see side bar).

○ *example:*

### FEBRUARY

| S | M | T | W | T | F | S |
|---|---|---|---|---|---|---|
|   |   |   | 1 | 2 | 3 | 4 |
| 5 | 6 | 7 | 8 | 9 | 10 | 11 |
| 12 | 13 | 14 | 15 | 16 | 17 | 18 |
| 19 | 20 | (21) | (22) | (23) | (24) | (25) |
| 26 | 27 | 28 |   |   |   |   |

*This chart indicates the date of the first day of the last menstrual period is February 21.*

## What if I am taking the "pill"?

If you are using any type of hormonal birth control, such as the birth control pill, implants, injections or a contraceptive patch or ring, you should allow yourself at least one normal menstrual cycle before trying to become pregnant. This rest period allows your body to return to normal. To protect yourself from pregnancy during this rest period, use a condom. If you become pregnant while taking the pill, stop immediately. Don't worry, there are no known ill effects to the baby if this happens.

## What about other forms of birth control?

There is no waiting period required after using spermicidal foams, jellies, condoms or a diaphragm, so you can try to become pregnant immediately.

If you have an intrauterine device (IUD) in place, you should have it removed before you try to get pregnant. If you accidentally do get pregnant with an IUD in place, you should have it taken out as soon as possible. Leaving an IUD in place during pregnancy is not a good idea. It can cause a miscarriage, an infection, or a premature birth. It is best to wait for at least one normal period to occur after the IUD is out before attempting to get pregnant. If you have an IUD in place and you suspect you may be pregnant, visit your health care provider for a pregnancy test to make sure. If possible, have the IUD removed. However, sometimes the IUD cannot be removed for medical reasons. If this is the case, you will be monitored carefully throughout your pregnancy for any problems it may cause.

---

### I DON'T HAVE TO MENTION THAT, DO I?

*It makes good sense to be direct and completely honest about your health and lifestyle.*

*Your health care team needs the whole picture to help you plan for a healthy pregnancy and birth.*

NUTRITION QUIZ

## NUTRITION QUIZ

*If you check any of these, you have special nutritional needs that you need to talk to your doctor about.*

- ☐ I am following a diet to lose weight.
- ☐ I "fast" on occasion.
- ☐ I take part in very strenuous exercise.
- ☐ I am overweight.
- ☐ I am underweight.
- ☐ I have an eating disorder.
- ☐ I don't like milk or other dairy products.
- ☐ I am a vegetarian.
- ☐ I have a history of low blood iron (anemia).
- ☐ I am a diabetic.
- ☐ I have a serious medical illness which affects what I can eat.
- ☐ I don't have enough money to buy the food I need.
- ☐ I have high cholesterol.
- ☐ I am always constipated.
- ☐ I do not eat fish.
- ☐ I do not eat red meat.

# What can I do to be healthy

### Nutrition

Eating well before you become pregnant will help your body meet the nutritional needs of your developing baby. Canada's Food Guide to Healthy Eating (reprinted on page 7) is a good guide to follow, both before and during your pregnancy, as it promotes eating a wide variety of wholesome foods every day. By establishing good eating habits now, you are also likely to find it easier to keep eating well throughout your pregnancy. For most women, following this guide will meet all of the nutritional requirements of pregnancy. In addition to eating a healthy, balanced diet, pregnant women should also eat often. Babies are constantly developing, so it's important for pregnant women to avoid long periods without eating (more than 12 hours). Ideally, pregnant women should try to eat three meals and three snacks spread throughout each day.

# Canada's Food Guide to Healthy Eating

OTHER FOODS

*Taste and enjoyment can also come from other foods and beverages that are not part of the 4 food groups. Some of these foods are higher in fat or calories, so use these foods in moderation.*

*Canada's Food Guide to Healthy Eating, Health Canada, 2005 © Minister of Public Works and Government Services Canada, 2005.*

## Different people need different amounts of food

The amount of food you need every day from the 4 food groups and other foods depends on your age, body size, activity level, whether you are male or female and if you are pregnant or breastfeeding. That's why the Food Guide gives a lower and higher number of servings for each food group. For example, young children can choose the lower number of servings, while male teenagers can go to the higher number. Most other people can choose servings somewhere in between.

## Other essential nutritional requirements

### Omega-3 fatty acids
These types of fats are considered "healthy" (your body needs them and so does your baby) and "essential" because your body cannot make them by itself. You must get omega-3 fatty acids through the food you eat. They have also been linked to health benefits for your heart, mental health, arthritis and prevention of preterm labour.

### Minerals and vitamins
Vitamin C, magnesium and zinc are important throughout your pregnancy and can even help reduce the risk of premature delivery. Pregnant women and their growing babies also need additional iron, protein, and B vitamins such as folic acid. These minerals and vitamins are found in red meat, chicken, fish, dry beans, eggs, nuts and fruit.

## Calcium

Calcium and vitamin D help to build strong bones and teeth for you and your baby. For pregnant women, the recommended daily intake of calcium is 1200-1500 mg, depending on her age. Canada's Food Guide to Healthy Eating recommends 3-4 servings of milk products each day of pregnancy. Pregnant women who do not take milk products may be at risk of not meeting their need in calcium, vitamin D and protein. If this is the case, speak to your health care provider about supplementation.

Milk products come top of the list as good sources of calcium – because they're rich in calcium, and the form of calcium they contain is well absorbed by the body. Other good, natural sources of easily-absorbed calcium include sardines and salmon with their bones, and also bok choy. Most other calcium-containing foods such as sesame seeds, nuts, dried beans and broccoli provide you with a lot less calcium, or provide it in a form that is less easily absorbed by the body.

---

**SOURCES OF OMEGA-3 FATTY ACIDS**

- Liquid oils such as olive, canola, sunflower and flaxseed.
- Salmon and other cold water fish such as sardines, halibut, bluefish, tuna and mackerel.
- Venison, buffalo.
- Leafy green vegetables.
- Omega-3 enriched eggs.

## Easy does it

By consuming the 3 to 4 daily servings of milk products recommended by Canada's Food Guide to Healthy Eating, a pregnant woman can easily meet her daily calcium needs. Each serving gives you about 300 mg of calcium.

Remember you need more than just calcium to maintain healthy bones. Other nutrients in foods in which calcium naturally occurs are often essential for bone maintenance. For example, milk products contain phosphorus, magnesium, vitamin D (milk only) and vitamin A, as well as protein that are important for healthy bones too. Canned salmon with its bones gives you vitamin D, phosphorus and protein, among other nutrients. If you want to build and maintain strong, healthy bones, it's always better to concentrate on foods that are natural sources of calcium, rather than turning to food supplements.

## Sources of calcium

| Food | Serving | | Calcium (mg) |
|---|---|---|---|
| **MILK PRODUCTS** | | | |
| Cheese, Parmesan, grated | 50 g | (2 oz) | 555 |
| Ricotta cheese, with partly skimmed milk | 125 ml | (1/2 cup) | 356 |
| Firm cheeses, such as Brick, Cheddar & Edam | 50 g | (2 oz) | 350 |
| Milk, partly skimmed, 2% b.f. | 250 ml | (1 cup) | 302 |
| Milk, chocolate, partly skimmed, 2% b.f. | 250 ml | (1 cup) | 301 |
| Yogourt, plain, <1% b.f. | 175 g | (3/4 cup) | 294 |
| Cheese, mozzarella, (52% water, 22.5% b.f.) | 50 g | (2 oz) | 269 |
| Feta cheese | 50 g | (2 oz) | 247 |
| Camembert cheese | 50 g | (2 oz) | 194 |
| Ice cream, vanilla, 11% b.f. | 125 ml | (1/2 cup) | 97 |
| Frozen yogourt | 125 ml | (1/2 cup) | 92 |
| Cottage cheese, creamed (4.5% b.f.) | 125 ml | (1/2 cup) | 71 |
| **FOODS PREPARED USING MILK PRODUCTS** | | | |
| Milk shake, vanilla, thick | 250 ml | (1 cup) | 364 |
| Soup made with whole milk | 250 ml | (1 cup) | 189 |
| Vanilla or chocolate pudding | 125 ml | (1/2 cup) | 152 |
| **OTHER FOODS** | | | |
| Tofu (made with calcium sulphate) | 1 serving | | 961 |
| Nuts, almonds, dried, unblanched | 60 ml | (1/4 cup) | 89 |
| Bok choy, cooked | 125 ml | (1/2 cup) | 84 |
| Orange, Florida, raw | 1 fruit (6.8 cm dia) | | 65 |
| Beans, lima, canned, solids and liquid | 125 ml | (1/2 cup) | 37 |
| Soybeans, mature seeds, sprouted, steamed | 125 ml | (1/2 cup) | 29 |
| Figs, dried, uncooked | 2 figs | | 27 |
| **LESS IMPORTANT SOURCES OF CALCIUM** | | | |
| Seeds, sesame seeds, roasted and toasted | 60 ml | | 376 |
| Beverage, soy, fluid, enriched | 250 ml | (1 cup) | 319 |
| Kale, frozen, boiled, drained | 125 ml | (1/2 cup) | 95 |
| Broccoli, frozen, chopped, unprepared | 125 ml | (1/2 cup) | 46 |

Source: Health Canada, Canadian Nutrient File, 2005

## Folic acid quiz

*If you are planning a pregnancy and you check any box below, you should talk to your doctor about folic acid.*

☐ I have epilepsy.

☐ I have anemia.

☐ I am an insulin-dependent diabetic.

☐ I have already had a pregnancy in which the baby had a neural tube defect.

☐ I take more than 0.4 mg of folic acid daily, without a doctor's advice.

☐ I have a close relative who was born with a neural tube defect.

## Folic acid

Folic acid is a vitamin that has been proven to help prevent neural tube birth defects such as spina bifida. These birth defects cause abnormal development of a baby's spinal cord or brain. These defects develop between the third and fourth week of pregnancy, in many cases before the woman even realizes she is pregnant. For this reason, taking 0.4-1 milligram (mg) of folic acid daily is recommended at least three months before becoming pregnant and throughout pregnancy in order to prevent neural tube defects. Women considered to be at a higher risk (see folic acid quiz) may sometimes benefit from taking higher doses, and should discuss this with their health care provider.

*Note: Addition of folic acid to white flour and pasta products labelled "enriched" became mandatory as of November 1998. This mandatory fortification will add approximately 100 µg (0.1 mg) of folic acid to the average woman's diet every day.*

*Source: Health Canada, Canadian Nutrient File, 1997 Visit the website at www.hc-sc.gc.ca/nutrition*

## Dietary sources of folic acid
*(based on usual serving size)*

**EXCELLENT SOURCE OF FOLIC ACID**
*(55 µg (MICROGRAMS) OR MORE)*

cooked fava, kidney, pinto, roman, soy, and white beans; chickpeas, lentils
cooked spinach, asparagus
romaine lettuce
orange juice, canned pineapple juice
sunflower seeds

**GOOD SOURCE OF FOLIC ACID**
*(33 µg (MICROGRAMS) OR MORE)*

cooked lima beans
corn, bean sprouts, cooked broccoli, green peas, Brussels sprouts, beets
orange
honeydew melon
raspberries, blackberries
avocado
roasted peanuts
wheat germ

**SOURCE OF FOLIC ACID**
*(11 µg (MICROGRAMS) OR MORE)*

cooked carrots, beet greens, sweet potato, snow peas, summer or winter squash, rutabaga, cabbage, cooked green beans
cashews, roasted peanuts, walnuts
eggs
strawberries, banana, grapefruit, cantaloupe
whole wheat or white bread
pork kidney
breakfast cereals
milk, all types

## What is anemia?

Hemoglobin is a substance found in the blood that transports oxygen from your lungs to other parts of your body and to your developing baby. Anemia means that a person has lower levels of hemoglobin in his or her blood. During pregnancy, a woman may develop anemia because of low levels of iron in her body. It can affect your energy levels, your exercise tolerance and your ability to provide oxygen to you and your baby.

Your health care provider can perform a blood test to determine if your hemoglobin level is normal (between 110-112 g/L). Because iron deficiency is common in pregnant women, health care providers often advise all pregnant women to take iron supplements during pregnancy.

### Sources of iron in your diet

*MILLIGRAMS (MG) OF IRON FOUND*
*IN EACH 100 GRAM PORTION*

*EXCELLENT SOURCES:*
*Liver (8.8 mg)*

*GOOD SOURCES:*
*Beef (3.1-3.9 mg),  Veal (3.2-3.6 mg)*

*SOURCES:*
*Lamb (2.0 mg), Chicken (1.3 mg), Pork (1.1 mg)*

*OTHER SOURCES OF IRON INCLUDE:*
*egg yolk, legumes, tofu,*
*dark green vegetables (spinach, broccoli, peas)*
*and dried fruits*

### AM I AT RISK FOR ANEMIA?

- *I have been told I have "low" hemoglobin or anemia before.*

- *I have a history of heavy periods.*

- *I do not eat red meat.*

- *I have a chronic illness.*

- *I have a family history of anemia.*

*If you answered yes to any of the above statements, speak to your health care provider.*

## Do I need to take vitamins?

Prenatal vitamins contain many important and beneficial vitamins and minerals, including folic acid. Depending on your diet, additional supplements of iron or calcium may be needed. However, it's important to understand that excess vitamins can be harmful, so you should consult your health care provider before you take any supplements. He or she may suggest getting further help or advice from a dietician.

## Nutrition quiz

Use this chart to check your eating habits for one week and compare them to the recommendations of Canada's Food Guide for Healthy Eating. Use this as a guide to eating for your pregnancy. Place an 'X' for each serving you have eaten during the day.

|  | Grain Products 5-12 servings | Fruits and Vegetables 5-10 servings | Milk 3-4 servings | Meats and Alternatives 2-3 servings |
|---|---|---|---|---|
| Day 1 |  |  |  |  |
| Day 2 |  |  |  |  |
| Day 3 |  |  |  |  |
| Day 4 |  |  |  |  |
| Day 5 |  |  |  |  |
| Day 6 |  |  |  |  |
| Day 7 |  |  |  |  |

## Remember

**Grain products:**
Includes bread, pasta, rice, cereal and other grains.
Choose whole grain products for best nutritional value.

**Fruits and vegetables:**
Choose fruit and dark green vegetables often.

**Meat and alternatives:**
Include a serving of this group at each meal.
Include one serving of fish each week.

**Essential fatty acids:**
Include 1-2 teaspoons of vegetable oil daily (i.e. used during cooking
or on a salad).

## Exercise

You don't need the muscular strength and endurance of a triathlete to
have a successful pregnancy, but being in generally good condition before
you conceive will help you feel your best throughout your pregnancy.

If you are already active, ask about continuing your sports or workout
activities safely. As your pregnancy progresses, your whole body is
affected, and you may be more prone to injury. For example, you will
need to limit high-impact activities and those that raise the body's core
temperature.

If you have been inactive and would like to get in shape now, begin
gradually. Try regular brisk walking, swimming, or other activities that
will strengthen your heart and lungs and tone your muscles. You can read
more about exercise during pregnancy in Chapter Two.

## Work

Women planning a pregnancy should take all recommended precautions when they must work with chemicals, solvents, fumes, and radiation. If you are already pregnant, your health care provider may advise you to avoid any contact at all with some of these workplace hazards.

Shift work, very strenuous work, or long working hours and commuting times can sometimes lead to miscarriage, or a small or premature baby. You can read more about what is considered strenuous work during pregnancy in Chapter Three.

## Smoking

A clearly proven link exists between smoking in pregnancy and small or premature babies. There is also a great deal of evidence suggesting that infants and children are harmed by secondhand smoke. If you or your partner smokes, an excellent way to prepare for being a parent is to stop smoking now.

If you are already pregnant, studies show that if you quit smoking before you reach your 16th week, there is less chance that your baby will be born too early or too small. Some researchers say your baby can still benefit greatly even if you quit smoking as late as 32 weeks into your pregnancy. As well, studies seem to indicate that you can increase your baby's birth weight by drastically cutting down how much you smoke during your pregnancy. Ideally, if you are thinking about having a baby, you should try to quit smoking before you conceive.  This way, your baby will reap the most health benefits. However, it is important to remember that there are health benefits to quitting at any time, even after your child is born.

If you do smoke, it's important to understand the risks of having a small or premature baby. Unfortunately, some women may mistakenly believe that the risk is minimal, or may even feel that a small baby is better as it will be easier to deliver. However, babies born too early and underweight are known to have a harder time adjusting to life outside the uterus. They are

- *My baby will get more oxygen from me.*
- *My baby will have less chance of breathing problems after she is born.*
- *My baby will be more likely to be a normal weight when he is born.*
- *My baby will be less likely to be born early.*
- *I will breathe better and have more energy.*
- *I will save money.*
- *I will feel good about myself for making a healthy decision for me and my baby.*

also more likely to have problems sleeping and eating, and are more prone to illness. If you are a smoker, you may smoke as a relief from stress—a cigarette is a reward, a break, a way to feel calm. It may be hard for you to find better ways to give yourself a break, but there is support available. (See page 40 for ways to relieve stress).

Be honest when you talk about your smoking habits. Ask about programs in your community that can help you to quit successfully. You may consider using a nicotine patch if you have tried other methods without much success.

*Make up your mind to quit, believe you can do it, take steps to change your behaviours and get help!*

*There are many resources in your community to help you quit smoking.*

### Smoking - Resources to Help You Quit

| | |
|---|---|
| Physicians for a Smoke-Free Canada | http://www.smoke-free.ca/Y2Quit |
| The Lung Association | http://www.on.lung.ca/getontrack/getontrack.html |
| Centres for Disease Control Tobacco and Information Source | http://www.cdc.gov/tobacco/quit/canquit.htm |
| Health Canada's e-Quit webpage | http://www.hc-sc.gc.ca/hecs-sesc/tobacco/quitting/e-quit/index.html |
| Health Canada's inventory of cessation programs | http://www.hc-sc.gc.ca/hecs-sesc/tobacco/quitting/index.html |
| Webpage dedicated to smoking cessation for pregnant women | http://www.pregnets.org/ |
| Alberta Alcohol and Drug Abuse Commission | http://tobacco.aadac.com/ |

## I CAN QUIT SMOKING!

### WHY?

- *I want to be in the best health for my pregnancy.*

- *I want my baby to have the best chance at being healthy.*

### HOW?

- *I will change some of my behaviour patterns.*

- *If I smoke after meals, I will get up after a meal and go for a walk.*

- *If I smoke when I am stressed, I will call a friend, listen to music or take a bath.*

### WHAT ABOUT OTHERS AROUND ME?

- *Ask others not to smoke around you.*

- *Go to non-smoking areas when you are out.*

## Do you have an alcohol problem?

- *Have you ever felt you should cut down on your drinking?*

- *Have people annoyed you by criticizing your drinking?*

- *Have you ever felt bad or guilty about your drinking?*

- *Have you ever had a drink first thing in the morning to steady your nerves or to get rid of a hangover?*

*If you answered yes to any of the above questions, talk to your health care provider.*

## Alcohol

Drinking alcohol during pregnancy can cause serious birth defects. Alcohol-related birth defects can range from learning disabilities and personality disorders to poor growth and development, and deformities of the face and brain. Just how harmful will a mother's drinking be? Mostly, it depends on her own health, how much she drinks and when.  Because of these serious health risks, most experts suggest that women should avoid alcohol altogether, throughout pregnancy.

No thanks, my baby's too young to drink

### Alcohol is harmful to my baby

Fetal alcohol spectrum disorder (FASD) describes a group of abnormalities of babies whose mothers had a history of drinking alcohol during their pregnancy. These babies may be smaller in weight and length. Despite good medical care, they may not catch up to normal babies. They may have small heads, heart defects, and poor control over their muscles. They sometimes show abnormalities of the face, limbs, and joints. They usually have some degree of cognitive delay and/or behavioural problems, including hyperactivity, extreme nervousness, and a poor attention span.

As children with fetal alcohol spectrum disorder grow up, they tend to have behavioural problems, learning problems in school, and trouble concentrating.

### For more information about FASD:

*Contact the Canadian Centre on Substance Abuse at 1-800-559-4514 or visit their website at www.ccsa.ca, or call the Motherisk Alcohol and Substance Use Helpline at 1-877-327-4636 or visit www.motherisk.org*

## Street drugs

It is important to understand that using street (illegal) drugs at any time during a pregnancy may cause damage to a developing baby. If used regularly, some of these drugs can even cause a baby to be born with an addiction. Babies born to mothers who use illegal drugs are usually smaller, tend to be more irritable and fussy, and may have brain damage that will affect their ability to learn.

If you are using illegal drugs, you need to stop before you get pregnant. If you have become pregnant while still using drugs, tell your health care provider. He needs to know about this, because you may need extra support and special care during pregnancy.

## Your medical history

Some illnesses or conditions a woman may have, or may have had in the past, can affect the outcome of her pregnancy. Women who have serious medical conditions, such as heart problems, diabetes, high blood pressure, or epilepsy, may need to be followed closely throughout their pregnancy by a specialist in that field. Overweight women should be tested for diabetes.

If you, your partner, or another close relative has one of the diseases that run in families such as muscular dystrophy, hemophilia, cystic fibrosis, Tay-Sachs disease, or beta-thalassemia discuss this with your doctor. She may refer you to a geneticist (a specialist in the field of heredity).

## Medication

Almost all medicines, including prescription and non-prescription drugs, can cross through the placenta and into a growing baby. Very few medicines are known to cause any harm to a newly forming baby, although most have not been studied to rule out this possibility. Drugs that have been shown

PRESCRIPTION AND
NON-PRESCRIPTION DRUGS,
HERBS AND VITAMINS YOU TAKE.

drug/herb/vitamin

amount taken

how often

how long

drug/herb/vitamin

amount taken

how often

how long

drug/herb/vitamin

amount taken

how often

how long

to cause harm usually do so within the first few weeks of pregnancy, when the baby's main body systems are still forming. Ideally, you should avoid using non-prescription drugs, including herbal products, while trying to conceive and during pregnancy. As a rule, talk to your health care provider before using any kind of drug, herb, plant or home remedy. He will know or can find out about current research into the safety of these products.

If you would like more information about toxic substances that may harm your baby, talk to the team at the Motherisk Program at the Hospital for Sick Children in Toronto by calling (416) 813-6780 or visit www.motherisk.org

If you are planning a pregnancy and have a condition that requires you to take prescription medication, it is very important to talk about it with your health care provider. Preferably, you should do this before you get pregnant. You may have to change the type of drug you take to one that cannot cross through the placenta and cannot harm your baby. If the prescription cannot be changed, you may be advised to reduce your dosage or stop using the drug altogether during your pregnancy, provided it is safe to do so.

### German measles (rubella)

In the late 1960s, a vaccine was developed to protect people against German measles (rubella) and it has been routinely given to all preschool children ever since. The main reason for the development of a vaccine was to prevent infection during pregnancy, which can result in serious birth defects for a baby. Today, most women are immune to rubella by the time they reach their childbearing years, either because they have been vaccinated or because they have developed protective antibodies after being exposed to the disease.

Your blood will be tested for antibodies that show you are protected against rubella. If you do not have these antibodies, you may need to be vaccinated. It is best to be vaccinated at least three months before becoming pregnant.

## MY MEDICAL HISTORY

*Check those that apply to you:*
- ☐ *Problems with an anesthetic.*
- ☐ *Operations.*

*Please list all operations:*

_____

_____

_____

- ☐ *Blood transfusion in the year _____.*
- ☐ *High cholesterol.*
- ☐ *Problems with my heart.*
- ☐ *High blood pressure.*
- ☐ *Diabetes.*
- ☐ *Problems with blood clots in my legs or in my lungs.*
- ☐ *A seizure-related disorder (epilepsy).*
- ☐ *Problems with my kidneys or bladder.*
- ☐ *Serious infection in the past.*

*Infectious diseases I have had:*

_____

_____

_____

- ☐ *A history of mental health problems.*
- ☐ *Problems getting pregnant.*
- ☐ *Allergies.*

## MY FAMILY'S MEDICAL HISTORY

*List anyone in your family, including your parents, brothers, sisters, grandparents, and children, who has any of the following medical conditions and describe the condition.*

*Diabetes*

_____

_____

*A hereditary disorder*

_____

_____

*High blood pressure*

_____

_____

*A deformity*

_____

_____

*Twins, triplets, or more*

_____

_____

*Other problems you think may be serious*

_____

_____

_____

19

TOLL-FREE HELP LINE ABOUT HIV
IN PREGNANCY

*Motherisk's toll-free HIV Healthline (1-888-246-5840) offers confidential counselling to Canadian women, their families, and health care providers about the risk of HIV and HIV treatment in pregnancy. This program also helps HIV specialists and community groups across Canada work together to help establish the safety or risk of HIV treatments.*

## Lifestyle and sexual history

You may feel uncomfortable with questions about your sexual habits, but, as with drug use, these questions are asked to help reduce risks to your baby.

If you have ever had sex without using a condom, particularly if you have had more than one sexual partner, you may have been exposed to a sexually transmitted disease, such as genital herpes, genital warts, chlamydia, gonorrhea, syphilis, or the HIV virus (which causes AIDS).

Some sexually transmitted diseases (STD) are curable; some are not. Some need to be treated to reduce the risk of infecting the baby at birth. Depending on your lifestyle and sexual history, certain tests can help you plan your prenatal care. HIV testing is now being offered to all women who are pregnant, and those thinking about getting pregnant, because there is effective treatment available for HIV-positive mothers to reduce the chances of giving their babies the virus. Women who live with a disease that comes back again and again, such as genital herpes or genital warts, can still have a normal pregnancy. Sometimes, particularly around the time of the baby's birth, these mothers may need special care. Visit www.sexualityandu.ca for more information on STDs.

## If you have been pregnant before

You will be asked about your past pregnancies and whether you had any problems during the months you were pregnant, during labour and delivery, or after birth. Knowledge of complications in past pregnancies can alert your health care provider to try to prevent them from happening again. You can still have a normal, healthy pregnancy. It is again very important to give as complete an obstetrical history as possible, in case you are going to need special care.

| I have been pregnant before | | | |
|---|---|---|---|
| | 1st | 2nd | 3rd |
| Date | | | |
| Name of hospital | | | |
| Hours in labour | | | |
| Delivery type | | | |
| Complications | | | |
| Boy/girl | | | |
| Birth weight | | | |

## Visit your health care provider before you get pregnant

If you are planning a pregnancy, book a checkup with your health care provider to make sure you are in good health and practicing a healthy lifestyle. You will be asked about your medical history, your family, any medications you may take, your diet, your past pregnancies, your sexual history and the kind of work you do.

If all goes well during this visit, you probably won't need to see your health care provider again until you suspect you are pregnant.

When planning your family, it is also important to learn as much as you can about pregnancy and childbirth. Studies have shown that women who learn about pregnancy are the most likely to have a satisfying childbirth experience. These women felt the information they learned helped them to be more in control of their pregnancy and childbirth, and so they felt more fulfilled with the experience. In one study, women who received prenatal education needed less pain-controlling medication during their labour, which suggests that they either had less pain or were better able to cope with the pain they had. More importantly, another study suggests that women were more likely to carry their babies to full term when they were made aware of the different risk factors that can cause premature births (page 52).

As you plan your family, remember that you play an important role in ensuring a healthy pregnancy and a healthy baby. Receiving regular prenatal care and keeping yourself healthy and informed are all excellent steps to help give your baby the best of healthy beginnings.

## RECORDING MY PROGRESS

Date:

Blood pressure:

Weight:

## THINGS TO DISCUSS WITH MY HEALTH CARE PROVIDER:

☐ Concerns with my diet.

☐ The kind of work that I do.

☐ Quitting smoking.

☐ Concerns with alcohol or drugs.

☐ My medical history.

☐ My family history.

☐ Exercise.

Other concerns:

# My pregnancy journal
# My health before pregnancy

NUTRITION QUIZ RESULTS:

| | | | |
|---|---|---|---|
| I follow Canada's Food Guide | Yes / No | I am taking folic acid | Yes / No |
| I have enough calcium in my diet | Yes / No | I have sources of vitamin C, magnesium, zinc and omega-3 fatty acids in my diet. | Yes / No |
| I get enough iron from my diet | Yes / No | | |

# Well begun: the first trimester

## WHAT IS A TRIMESTER?

*A trimester is a three-month time period, and is the term used for each of the three parts of a full-term pregnancy, which lasts approximately nine months. The countdown begins at conception, and the first trimester ends at about 13 weeks. The second trimester ends at 25 to 26 weeks and the third extends from about 26 to 40 weeks.*

## WHEN IS MY DUE DATE?

*The approximate date your baby will be born (your due date) is calculated by counting nine calendar months plus seven days from the first day of your last menstrual period. About 85 percent of babies arrive within a week before or a week after their due date.*

*Your first trimester lasts three months, until about your 13th week of pregnancy. It is a time of rapid fetal growth and development, and the time when your body adjusts to pregnancy. The choices you make about your health, diet, and lifestyle from now on will affect both you and your unborn baby.*

*Finding out you are pregnant can be one of the most exciting moments in your life, especially if you have been planning and hoping to become pregnant for some time. However, first weeks of your pregnancy may bring anxiety along with joy. What's happening to my body? What if the baby is not all right? Am I going to feel like this for nine months?*

*This anxiety is perfectly normal, but try not to worry. For one thing, you're off to a great start by using this handbook and learning as much as you can about pregnancy.*

## Your changing body

By the end of the third month, your body will have undergone dramatic changes. You may not look very pregnant yet, but you probably feel quite different. High levels of pregnancy hormones are responsible for almost all the changes your body will go through. From the moment of fertilization, your body begins to build a safe place for your baby to grow. This building process is complex, energy consuming, and the reason you feel so tired in your early months.

Your uterus slowly enlarges from the size of a kiwi to the size of a grapefruit. Your milk glands are now developing, your breasts feel fuller, heavier, and tender. Your heart works harder now because your body has produced extra blood for the growing placenta, and to provide oxygen and nutrients to your baby. You may become more aware of your breathing or feel breathless as a result of hormone changes. Usually, your menstrual cycle will stop. If you have any bleeding during pregnancy, check with your health care provider.

## Your developing baby

By the end of this trimester, your baby will be 13 weeks old, about 9 cm long (3.5 inches) and weigh about 48 grams (1.7 ounces). At this stage, your baby will still have plenty of space to move freely and will be very active, although you won't be able to feel movement until later. The baby's body will now be fully formed, but still needs time to gain weight and for organs to mature.

At 13 weeks, the fingers and toes are developed. The bones are mostly soft cartilage but they are beginning to harden. The head still appears too large when compared to the rest of the body. There are signs of 32 tooth buds in the jaw. The heart beats about 140 times per minute. The lungs are developed and the baby "breathes" amniotic fluid. By 12 weeks the baby is already practicing to suck by pursing the lips, turning the head and swallowing amniotic fluid, which is then passed as urine.

## How often should I expect to visit my health care provider?

An appointment every 4-6 weeks is appropriate for the beginning of pregnancy. After 30 weeks, visits should occur every 2-3 weeks. After 36 weeks, you should see your health care provider every 1-2 weeks until you go into labour.

*The embryo develops rapidly during the first 8 weeks of pregnancy.*

### WHY DO I NEED TO GO TO THE DOCTOR? I FEEL FINE.

*Prenatal care is the medical care you will receive before your baby is born. Although almost all pregnancies progress normally and most babies are born healthy, studies show that women who have regular prenatal care have better pregnancy outcomes. Unless you have a concern that you would like to discuss sooner, set up your first prenatal visit before 12 weeks have passed since your last menstrual period.*

*Receiving proper prenatal care is an important part of making sure all goes well during your pregnancy. Regular prenatal checkups also let you become better acquainted with your doctor, and feel more comfortable in sharing concerns and asking questions.*

*With consistent prenatal care, your doctor can identify problems early in your pregnancy and take steps to try to prevent any harm from coming to you or your baby.*

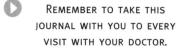
## Your first prenatal visit

Your first visit is usually more in-depth and longer than the rest. It may include a pregnancy test to confirm your pregnancy, an internal physical exam of your reproductive organs and pelvis, as well as a complete "checkup" of your whole body. Your health care provider will listen to your heart and check your blood pressure. Your height and weight will be measured.

Details about your medical and obstetrical history will be explored. If you saw your health care provider when you were planning to get pregnant, you may go over some of the same topics you discussed then. During this visit, your health care provider will also calculate your due date. This is usually done by calculating from the 1st day of your last menstrual period, so you should make sure that you have this date handy for your first visit.

Your health care provider knows how important it is for you to be well informed about your pregnancy and your developing baby. But office visits, even this first long one, may not cover every topic. That's why you will be encouraged to read education materials such as this handbook and to attend prenatal classes.

## What are all these tests for?

When you have your first prenatal visit, a number of laboratory tests are routinely recommended. These help predict risks to your health and that of your baby. They may include:

**Hemoglobin:** A hemoglobin test checks your blood to make sure it is able to carry enough iron and oxygen. (See page 11 – What is anemia?)

**Blood group and antibody screen:** This blood test checks to see what type of blood and Rh factor you have and looks for any unusual antibodies in your blood. (See blood group and Rh factor on the next page).

**Rubella titre:** This blood test checks to see if you have immunity to rubella (German measles). (See page 18 – German measles).

**Varicella (chicken pox):** If you have previously had chicken pox, your body will already have immunity and testing will not be required. If not, a test will be ordered to check for antibodies to this virus.

**Hepatitis B surface antigens:** A blood test to see if you have been exposed to hepatitis B (read more about hepatitis B on page 28).

**VDRL:** A blood test to screen for possible previous exposure to syphilis, a sexually transmitted disease.

**Urine test:** A test to check sugar and protein levels in your urine, and to see if you have a urinary tract infection (chronic urinary tract infections have been linked to an increased risk of premature labour).

**Pap test:** Pap tests are done to check for cancer of the cervix or conditions that could lead to cancer.

**HIV:** A blood test to check for a possible previous exposure to HIV, the virus that causes AIDS.

## Blood group and Rh factor

Your blood is one of four types: A, B, AB, or O. A person's blood type is determined by the type of "antigen" attached to the blood cells. An antigen is a protein that causes a response from your immune system (the system that protects you from infection). Type A blood has only A antigens attached to its blood cells. Type B blood has only B antigens. Type AB has both antigens. Type O blood has none.

### WHAT IS FIFTH DISEASE AND SHOULD I BE WORRIED?

*Fifth disease is a common viral illness caused by parvovirus B19. Because young children can contract this illness, pregnant mothers often can come in contact with it. The virus causes a mild illness in children, often with a red rash on the face, trunk and limbs. If a pregnant woman is exposed there are usually no serious complications. Over half of women have previously been infected and are immune. If infected, the mother may have fever, rash and joint pain but most women have no symptoms. In very rare cases, it can infect an unborn baby and cause illness or death.*

*If a pregnant woman is exposed to or develops signs of parvovirus infection, she should have her blood tested for antibodies to determine if she is immune. Certain women are at a higher risk of infection, including daycare workers, school teachers, and mothers of young children. Hand washing may help to decrease infection; however, there is no evidence that women reduce their risk of infection by leaving work. If you are pregnant and think you may have been exposed to this virus, talk to your health care provider.*

☐ *I have received a blood transfusion or blood products for a clotting disorder.*

☐ *I have had more than one sexual partner.*

☐ *I have injected drugs.*

☐ *I have shared needles when I injected drugs.*

☐ *I have handled blood or blood products at my job.*

☐ *I was born in Asia.*

*If you checked one or more boxes, you are at higher risk of having hepatitis B.*

▶ *If you have hepatitis B, your baby can be protected with vaccination.*

## What is Rh disease?

Another antigen that sometimes attaches to blood cells is called the Rh factor antigen. If your blood has this antigen, it is Rh positive. If your blood does not, it is Rh negative. Only 15 percent of the population is Rh negative. But, if you are Rh negative and the baby's father is Rh positive, your child might inherit his Rh factor rather than yours, making your baby Rh positive too. If an Rh-positive baby is growing inside an Rh-negative mother, the two blood types are not compatible. Should the mother's blood and the baby's blood mix, such as at birth or if bleeding occurs during pregnancy, the mother's body may react as if it had an allergy to the baby. The mother's body will begin to produce antibodies, which will fight the Rh-positive antigens in the baby's blood. This is called Rh disease.

### Rh disease is rare

This blood incompatibility may lead to serious illness or even death for the baby. With advances in modern medicine, this incompatibility is now preventable, and therefore seldom seen. If your blood test shows there is a need to prevent your body from forming antibodies, you will be given Rh-immune globulin (RhIg) when you are about 28 to 32 weeks pregnant and again after your baby is born, or at any time during pregnancy if bleeding occurs.

## Hepatitis B

Hepatitis is a viral infection that affects the liver. Hepatitis B can be sexually transmitted or passed to a baby during childbirth, and is the most serious type of hepatitis to have during pregnancy. One in every 250 people has this disease. It is more common in people who have recently emigrated from Asia. Many people have no symptoms and therefore don't realize they have it. They are called chronic carriers and can pass hepatitis B on to other people. A small percentage of chronic carriers go on to develop very serious and life-threatening liver disease.

Without treatment, about 50 percent of babies born to mothers who test positive for the hepatitis B virus get infected. This usually happens during the birth process or while breastfeeding. Without treatment, many of these babies will become chronic carriers as well, and a few may develop long-term health problems. To prevent this, babies born to mothers who test positive for hepatitis B are now treated soon after birth with a hepatitis B immune globulin, and also with the hepatitis B vaccine. Through these methods, 95 percent of these babies are prevented from being infected and from becoming carriers.

## HIV

The human immune deficiency virus (HIV) causes infections and diseases that harm a person's immune and nervous systems. As people become sicker with HIV infections, they may be diagnosed with AIDS (acquired immune deficiency syndrome). As symptoms of HIV may take five years or more to appear, many people with HIV are unaware they have it. HIV can be detected by testing a person's blood for presence of the virus.

The virus is found in an infected person's body fluids—semen, blood, vaginal secretions, and breast milk. Most commonly, the virus is spread from an infected person to a non-infected person during sex. However, the virus can also enter a person's bloodstream by way of a contaminated needle, so you are at risk if you share needles with an HIV-positive intravenous drug user. An infected mother can pass the virus on to her baby during pregnancy, delivery, or while breastfeeding. Very rarely, an HIV infection can occur from a blood transfusion.

### Take the test. Treatment is available.

*The number of women of childbearing age who are infected with HIV is increasing. Pregnant women can pass the virus to their unborn child or to their newborn via breast milk. Today there is treatment to help prevent this. Unless treated, many babies who are infected with HIV die within three years. That is why every woman who is pregnant, or thinking about becoming pregnant, should strongly consider being tested for HIV. Every pregnant woman in Canada is offered HIV testing during pregnancy.*

---

### DO I HAVE A LIFESTYLE THAT PUTS ME AT RISK FOR CONTRACTING A SEXUALLY TRANSMITTED DISEASE?

☐ *I have had multiple sexual partners.*

☐ *I have had sex with multiple partners, some of whom did not wear a condom.*

☐ *I use illegal drugs.*

☐ *I inject illegal drugs.*

☐ *I have a drinking problem.*

☐ *I participate in anal sex.*

*If you agree with any of these statements, you are at higher risk of having contracted a sexually transmitted disease, and should be tested for the presence of an STD (including AIDS).*

CHORIONIC VILLUS SAMPLING

AMNIOCENTESIS

ULTRASOUND

In Canada, this is no longer a high risk, as the blood supply is now carefully screened for the presence of disease.

You can reduce the likelihood of contracting HIV by limiting the number of sexual partners you have and asking questions about your partner's sexual history before you make love for the first time. Ideally, when you begin a new relationship, you should use a condom for at least six months. After two negative HIV tests by both parties, as long as neither of you has other lovers, you are probably safe to stop using condoms. If you use injection drugs, never share needles.

## Genetic screening

At your first prenatal visit, your health care provider may talk about genetic testing, unless you have already discussed the issues thoroughly at a pre-pregnancy visit.

Many factors determine whether you would benefit from genetic testing for fetal abnormalities early in your pregnancy. Your age, medical, obstetrical, and genetic histories are important. Any genetic disorders or birth defects your close relatives have will impact on your pregnancy.

If your family's medical history raises concerns, or if you are more than 35 years old, you should talk to your health care provider about testing.

In most provinces, some type of genetic screening is offered to all women. The type of testing varies according to the availability of screening programs in your area.

Testing may be done in one of two ways. One method tests all pregnant women for certain conditions (e.g. maternal serum screening (MSS)); the other offers specific testing to those identified as being at a high risk of giving birth to a child with birth defects.

## Types of Tests

### Maternal serum screening (MSS)

This is a blood test that measures substances in the blood called "markers." If these markers are present in a person's blood in higher levels, it may indicate a risk of certain birth defects such as Down's syndrome (chromosome problem) or neural tube defects (brain or spinal cord problems). MSS is a screening test, so it may give a result, which requires further testing. If MSS is offered in your area, there will be further reading material available to help you decide whether or not to undergo this testing.

### Chorionic villus sampling (CVS)

This test is performed when you are between 9 and 11 weeks pregnant. A needle is inserted into the uterus, either through the opening of the uterus (cervix) or through the abdomen. A small sample of special cells (chorionic villi) is taken from the placenta for testing.

### Amniocentesis

This test is done between your 15th and 16th week. A fine needle is inserted into the uterus via the abdomen. Ultrasound is used to help the doctor find a safe place to insert the needle. A sample of the amniotic fluid that surrounds the baby is taken for testing.

### Ultrasound

This test is a screen for the entire baby. It creates a picture of your baby on a computer screen, using sound waves. Ultrasound is now routinely used to see the baby's position and how well it is growing, to discover where the placenta is attached to the uterus, to count the fetal heart rate, to see how many babies there are, and to check for some abnormalities. Ultrasound is also used to confirm your baby's due date.

### Nuchal cord translucency

This is a special type of ultrasound that may be offered. It measures an area around the baby's neck. Similar to maternal serum screening, it is a screening test, which can indicate a likelihood of certain abnormalities.

ULTRASOUND

*None of the available tests are 100 percent accurate and none test for all possible conditions.*

*Talk to your health care provider about which testing is available and recommended for you. Ultimately, it is your decision whether or not to go ahead with genetic testing.*

## Detecting genetic disorders and birth defects

*If you, one of your relatives, or your child had a birth defect, try to find out the name of the disease and fill in this chart. It can be helpful to mention this to your doctor before your 9th week of pregnancy. These disorders can sometimes be detected using specialized tests that will require a referral to a genetics specialist.*

| | |
|---|---|
| Congenital heart defect | Tay-Sachs disease |
| Spina bifida | Cystic fibrosis |
| Anencephaly | Thalassemia |
| Cleft palate | Hemophilia |
| Clubfoot | Muscular dystrophy |
| Huntington's disease | Fragile x syndrome |
| Born with extra fingers or toes | Down syndrome |
| Sickle cell disease | Other |

## Who will deliver my baby?

Health care providers increasingly work in groups to provide 24-hour care all year around. In Canada, obstetricians, family physicians, midwives and nurses provide maternity care in a normal pregnancy. However, complicated cases are usually referred to an obstetrician. It is best to discuss your individual situation with your health care provider.

All the information gathered during your pregnancy will be recorded on a special prenatal form. That way, any nurse, doctor, midwife, or other health care provider who reviews your prenatal record can be brought up to date about your pregnancy.

## Prenatal classes

Many thousands of women and their families take part in prenatal classes every year. Women report feeling more confident when they understand the changes pregnancy brings. Prenatal classes bring women and their families together, giving them a chance to share their experiences, wisdom, and feelings. Certainly, learning about pregnancy helps women to make informed decisions about their pregnancy and childbirth.

At one time, prenatal classes focused on the stages of labour and pain control during delivery. Today's classes still deal with these topics, but they also cover prenatal nutrition, parenting skills, signs of problems, exercise during pregnancy, and sexual relations during pregnancy. Classes are particularly helpful to women who are having their first baby and to young women who are pregnant during their teen years. Expectant fathers can learn about their changing relationship with their partners and their new role as a parent. Children can learn to be prepared for the arrival of a new brother or sister.

LIST NUMBERS FOR DATES, LOCATIONS, AND TIMES OF PRENATAL CLASSES:

**Avoid smells** *that make you feel
nauseated such as cooking odours
or perfume. Get your partner to
prepare meals if possible.*

**Eat whatever food you want**
*that looks and smells appealing and
that relieves your nausea.*

**Avoid warm places**
*feeling hot can add to nausea.*

**Sniffing fresh lemons or ginger,**
*drinking lemonade, or eating
watermelon slices seems to help.*

**Eating salty potato chips** *has
been found to help settle stomachs
enough to eat a meal.*

**Acupressure or acupuncture
treatment** *has been beneficial to
many women to help control nausea
and vomiting.*

**Avoid spicy, fried or fatty** *foods
and caffeine.*

**Avoid** *brushing your teeth
immediately after meals.*

If you are more comfortable learning in a language other than English, you may be able to find prenatal classes that are offered in different languages and will take into consideration the participants' ethnic and cultural backgrounds. There are often classes for teens.

Some communities offer postnatal classes to help families adjust to their new baby by exploring issues such as breastfeeding, getting back into shape, sexuality after pregnancy, and normal infant growth and development.

If you are interested in taking part in prenatal or postnatal classes, ask your health care provider where to sign up in your area.

## Common discomforts in early pregnancy

### Nausea and vomiting

The cause of "morning sickness" is still not known. Usually it occurs during the first three or four months of pregnancy, but it can linger. You may feel nauseated at any time during the day or night and when your stomach is empty.

For most women, the feeling of nausea and episodes of vomiting reduce at some point during the day allowing them to feel hungry again and to keep food down. However, one percent of pregnant women in Canada (about 4000 women per year) will suffer from such severe nausea and vomiting that the lack of foods, fluids, and nutrients may be harmful to their health and the well-being of their baby.

If left untreated, severe nausea and vomiting can lead to weight loss and aggravation of electrolyte imbalance. Electrolytes are substances that play an important role in making sure that the body works normally. Imbalances in the level of electrolytes such as sodium, calcium, chloride, magnesium, and phosphate can lead to health problems for pregnant women and their babies.

For these reasons, it is important to talk to a health care provider if you have nausea and vomiting during pregnancy. You may also consult the Society of Obstetricians and Gynaecologists of Canada website at www.sogc.org

## Getting help for morning sickness

WHAT CAN YOU DO?

- When you first wake up, eat a few crackers and then rest for 15 minutes before getting out of bed.
- Get up slowly and do not lie down right after eating.
- Eat small meals or snacks often so your stomach does not feel empty.
- Drink small amounts of fluids frequently during the day. Avoid drinking fluids during meals.
- Pregnant women usually need more sleep in the first three months of pregnancy. Try napping during the day.
- You may need to take time off work and get help and support from friends and family.

### Medication for nausea and vomiting

It is important to stay away from over-the-counter medications when you're pregnant. However, there is a safe and effective prescription medication that can help. Diclectin (a combination of vitamin $B_6$ and an antihistamine called doxylamine) is the only medication approved by Health Canada for the treatment of nausea and vomiting in pregnancy.  It has been proven to cause no harmful effects on babies and is considered safe and effective. Call the Motherisk Program at (416) 813-6780 for more information or visit www.motherisk.org

*For further information:  If you have access to the World Wide Web, visit the Motherisk Program's website at www.motherisk.org*

---

HOW TO GET OUT OF CHANGING TIGGER'S LITTER BOX

*Toxoplasmosis is a disease caused by a microscopic parasite that lives in a host animal and is passed on to other animals through feces. Up to half of the world's human population has been exposed to the parasite, but it is rare for an adult to have any symptoms. There is a small risk of birth defects in a baby born to a mother exposed to the parasite during her pregnancy.*

*Just to be on the safe side, avoid eating undercooked meat or chicken when you are pregnant, and wear rubber gloves when you handle raw meat or chicken. If you have a cat, try to have someone else change the litter box. If you must do it, wear gloves, avoid inhaling the dust, and wash your hands well afterwards. Also, you should avoid digging in a garden or lawn where cats may have gone to the bathroom.*

## Protecting the unborn child*

*The best way to protect an unborn child in a collision is to protect the mother. Pregnant women should always wear the lap and shoulder seat belt. The lap belt should be snug and low over the pelvic bones and not against the soft stomach area. The shoulder belt should be worn across the chest. Worn properly, the seat belt will not harm the baby.*

* Adopted from Transport Canada's website: http://www.tc.gc.ca/roadsafety/tp/tp13511/tips.htm

### Tender, painful breasts

The most important thing you can do is get a good support bra and wear it all the time, even at night. Make sure it fits properly and that it has full, rounded cups with wide, non-elastic shoulder straps. Warm compresses sometimes help, and if your nipples are sore, try applying some moisturizing cream.

### Tiredness

Two things cause the unusual tiredness many women feel during the first few months. First, your metabolism has increased, which is very energy consuming. Second, one of the pregnancy hormones (progesterone) has a sedative effect. The best advice is not to fight it. Pay attention to your body when you feel you need rest, or even a nap. Many women who "never nap" find themselves suddenly very ready for a little daytime rest. If it is possible at your workplace, try to find a quiet place to put your feet up and close your eyes when you have breaks. If this is impossible, plan to lie down as soon as you get home from work.

### Headaches

Headaches are quite common during pregnancy and they are not usually cause for alarm. However, if you have headaches that are constant, very severe, cause blurred vision, nausea, or spots to appear in front of your eyes, you should contact your health care provider.

If you have a headache, try lying down in a dark, cool room. Place a cool cloth on your forehead. Ask your partner for a neck and back massage. You can also try eating small meals often. Sometimes the headache is related to low blood sugar, especially if you are feeling nauseated and don't feel like eating. Discuss use of any pain medication with your health care provider.

### Frequent urination

Have you found yourself heading for the bathroom a lot more often lately? It is normal in early pregnancy to frequently have the urge to urinate. This is caused by the growing uterus putting pressure on your bladder and the increased amount of urine being produced by your kidneys. You may feel as though your bladder is very full but, when you go to the washroom, you find you only pass a little urine. Sometimes this pressure causes urine to leak out when you move or cough. Kegel exercises may help (see page 46). If you feel any pain when you urinate, you need to have this checked out. You may have an infection.

### Bleeding

Some women have some harmless spotting in the early months of pregnancy and go on to deliver healthy babies, but if you have any bleeding at all you should take it seriously, as it may be a sign of possible miscarriage. Get in touch with your health care provider.

Losing a baby through miscarriage happens in about 15 percent of pregnancies. A miscarriage seems to be the body's way of ending a pregnancy that is not developing normally. A miscarriage will usually not prevent a woman from having a normal pregnancy in the future, but it is best to wait at least one menstrual cycle before trying again.

### Fainting

Feeling faint is common during pregnancy and is probably explained by the combination of increased hormone levels, your changing circulatory system, and low blood sugar levels. If you feel lightheaded, try eating something sweet. Eating small nutritious meals and snacks between meals can help alleviate this. When you feel faint, sit down and put your head between your knees. Loosen any tight clothing and place a cool, wet cloth on your forehead or the back of your neck. If the feeling persists, call your health care provider.

> PREGNANT WOMEN SHOULD INCREASE THEIR CALORIC INTAKE BY ABOUT 100 CALORIES PER DAY IN THE 1ST TRIMESTER, BY 300 CALORIES PER DAY IN THE 2ND AND 3RD TRIMESTER AND 450 CALORIES PER DAY WHILE BREASTFEEDING.

> REMEMBER SPECIAL NEEDS *for calcium, iron, folic acid, essential fatty acids, minerals and vitamins. Refer to the nutrition section in Chapter One.*

ARE YOU SOMEONE WHO HAS GREATER NEEDS FOR CALORIES AND PROTEIN?

*I am having twins or multiples.*

*I am a teenager.*

*I am very physically active.*

*I have had a previous low birth weight baby weighing less than 5 1/2 pounds.*

*I am underweight.*

*I am undergoing emotional distress.*

## About weight gain

Researchers have not determined the exact amount of weight a woman should gain during pregnancy.

Most women gain somewhere between 11 and 16 kg (25-35 pounds). However, a woman can gain more or less than those amounts and still have a perfectly normal pregnancy and childbirth.

Eating a healthy, well-balanced diet is much more important than counting calories and worrying about whether you are gaining too much or too little weight. Follow Canada's Food Guide to Healthy Living (page 7), maintain an active lifestyle and allow your appetite to guide your food intake and you will likely gain the right amount of weight for you. What we do know is that women should not diet during pregnancy, even if they are overweight before the pregnancy. Women who are underweight and teenagers in particular should eat heartily, properly, and often.

For more information about nutrition and pregnancy, see Chapter One. If you have an Internet connection, try the links at the Motherisk website: www.motherisk.org

## About vitamin supplements

Prenatal vitamin supplements contain many of the extra vitamins required during pregnancy, such as folate and iron. Diets lacking in other essential foods (e.g. vegetarian or no-milk-product diets) may need further supplementation and you should discuss this with your health care provider. Nutrients are best obtained from eating healthy foods.

## About abuse

One in 12 women in Canada is a victim of physical violence. Physical abuse during pregnancy can cause serious injuries to the mother and cause her baby to be born too early or too small. Some unborn babies have died because of abuse suffered by their mothers.

If you are pregnant and a victim of physical abuse, you probably feel very alone. You need help now.

No one deserves to be abused. Sometimes, abuse in a family can leave a woman feeling embarrassed and ashamed, and that the abuse was her fault. If this is your situation, please ask for help. Talk to your health care provider, who will appreciate your courage and can help you find the community resources you will need.

If you would like more information about abuse, and places you can turn to for help, visit the website www.shelternet.ca

## Types of woman abuse

**Physical:** slapping, punching, kicking, biting, shoving, choking.

**Emotional or psychosocial:** intimidation, harassment, excessive jealousy, control, isolation, threats.

**Verbal:** constant criticism, blaming, false accusations, name calling, threats of violence towards a woman, people or things she cares about.

**Environmental:** making a woman afraid in her home by destroying property or possessions.

**Social:** isolating a woman from her family and friends.

**Financial:** preventing a woman from having control over money or expenditures, exploiting her economically.

**Sexual:** forced sexual activity.

**Religious or spiritual:** ridiculing a woman's beliefs, using beliefs to manipulate.

*Adopted from: Health Canada. A Handbook for Health and Social Service Professionals Responding to Abuse During Pregnancy. Prepared by Jamieson, Beals, Lalonde and Associates, Inc. Ottawa: Minister of Public Works and Government Services Canada, 1999.*

### ARE YOU IN AN ABUSIVE RELATIONSHIP?

☐ *Do you solve disagreements with fighting?*

☐ *Do you feel frightened by what your partner says or does?*

☐ *Have you ever been hit, pushed, shoved, or slapped by your partner?*

☐ *Has your partner ever been mean to you or made you feel worthless or stupid?*

☐ *Have you ever been forced to have sex against your will?*

*If you have answered yes to any of these questions, discuss this with your health care provider or someone who can help.*

WHEN THE ONE WHO LOVES YOU HURTS YOU.

CYCLE OF VIOLENCE

I'm sorry
Romance
Stage

Tension
Building

Explosive Event

## About stress and your support group

Everyone has some stress in their life but having too much stress is not healthy, particularly during pregnancy. Research has shown that stress in pregnant women may be associated with premature birth and low birth weight babies.

How much support you receive from the people around you can have a direct effect on how much stress you feel during your pregnancy. If you receive very little support, you may feel lonely and depressed.

Although pregnancy is a joyous time for most couples, the change and adjustments can sometimes cause strain within your relationship. Unexpected life events may increase your stress levels. If this happens to you, get help.

### Ways to reduce your stress

WOMEN WITH TOO MUCH STRESS NEED TO LEARN HEALTHY WAYS TO DEAL WITH IT.

1. Share the joys, challenges, and worries of pregnancy with someone close to you. This can make your pregnancy seem less stressful. If, for whatever reason, you don't have the support of your partner, try to spend time with other people you enjoy.

2. Attend prenatal classes and meet other women going through pregnancy. The breathing and concentration exercises taught for childbirth can help you relax now.

3. Get active. Exercise has been proven to lift the spirits and reduce stress.

4. Get enough sleep.

5. Learn other rest and relaxation techniques by reading books and listening to audiotapes, available in most public libraries.

6. Knowledge and preparation can reduce the anxiety you may be feeling about the birth itself. Working with your health care provider and support person to prepare a birth plan may help. Read about birthing plans on pages 75-81.

## Diabetes and pregnancy

Your body produces, in the pancreas, the substance insulin. Insulin is needed to make sure that sugar (glucose) is able to get inside your body's cells to produce energy. Without insulin, the glucose would remain in your blood. If too much glucose is in your bloodstream, you will have high blood glucose levels and no energy production in your cells.

Energy is needed to make all of your body organs work properly, including your lungs, brain, and your heart and blood vessels.

A mild diabetic has a pancreas that produces some insulin, but not enough to move all the glucose they need into their cells. These people are able to control their blood glucose levels by eating properly and by getting regular exercise to burn off the extra glucose. Some diabetics cannot produce any insulin in their pancreas at all, and must take insulin by injection in order for any glucose to reach the inside of their cells. Without insulin, a person cannot live.

Some women become diabetic during pregnancy. This is called gestational diabetes and is discussed in Chapter Three.

### If you have insulin-dependent diabetes

When a person's pancreas does not produce any insulin, he or she must get insulin from somewhere else in order to survive—most commonly synthetic insulin. This person is said to have Insulin Dependent Diabetes Mellitus (IDDM), also called Type I diabetes. They must test their blood glucose levels every day, and then inject the right amount of insulin to keep their blood glucose levels normal. For some people, having good control of their blood glucose levels is not always easy. When an insulin-dependent woman becomes pregnant, this challenge becomes even greater.

Good control of blood glucose levels is very important for a healthy pregnancy, especially in the month of conception and in the first trimester. Babies born to mothers whose blood glucose levels are not under tight control during their entire pregnancy may be unusually large (4.5 kg/ 10 lbs. or more) and hard to deliver, or they may have birth defects.

A diabetic woman should be followed by a health care professional team on a regular basis to make sure her blood sugar is well controlled.

## Dental health

New research has shown that pregnant women with tooth decay and gum disease are at higher risk for premature delivery.

## About sex

With pregnancy, many women experience a change in their levels of sexual desire, especially during this first trimester. Your hormones are making your breasts and vulva more sensitive, and this may make lovemaking more attractive. However, fatigue, nausea, and vomiting may make it the furthest thing from your mind. Don't worry—if you are in either camp, you have lots of company.

Some couples feel closer during this special time and continue to have enjoyable lovemaking until just before their baby is due. Other couples feel their relationship is strained as a result of all the changes taking place and find that sex is not as fulfilling during pregnancy. Your partner may be worried that having sex could harm the baby. If either of you is reluctant to make love, make time for other kinds of physical intimacy that may still appeal: cuddling, holding hands, massage, or bathing together, for example.

Usually, having intercourse will not harm the pregnancy in any way. However, your health care provider may advise you to avoid or limit intercourse if you have an infection, problems with bleeding, or problems with leaking amniotic fluid or the breaking of the amniotic sac. But that doesn't have to mean no lovemaking. If you feel like it, explore alternatives to vaginal sex, such as mutual masturbation or oral sex. Just a warning about oral sex—ask your partner to be careful not to blow any air into your vagina. Doing this could force air into your bloodstream and cause an air embolism that could be fatal to both you and your baby.

---

**DENTAL HEALTH IS IMPORTANT IN PREGNANCY.**

☐ *Do you have problems with your teeth or jaw?*

☐ *Are you brushing and flossing regularly?*

☐ *When was the last time you saw your dentist?*

*If you have tooth decay, sore or bleeding gums or have not seen your dentist in the last 6-12 months, make a dental appointment. It is both safe and important to visit a dentist during your pregnancy.*

## About exercise during pregnancy

There are different kinds of "workouts" that can be part of your daily routine, now that you are pregnant: aerobic exercise (with caution), strength training, relaxation techniques, and Kegel exercises.

### Aerobic exercise

Exercise that is strenuous enough to make your heart beat more quickly than when you are resting is called aerobic. It can include brisk walking, jogging, cycling, swimming, or team sports.

If you have been active before, you can probably continue with the same or a modified level of activity. But clear your exercise plans with your health care provider as early in your pregnancy as possible, so he or she can rule out any conditions that would make vigorous exercise risky.

So how can you tell if you are overexerting yourself? Try the "talk test." You should always be able to carry on a conversation during your workout.

If you get the green light from the health care provider, go for it. Walk, swim, or join a fitness class, especially one that is designed for pregnant women and new mothers. If you are in a regular aerobics class, speak to your instructor about avoiding routines that are high-impact, or that put stress on your lower back.

Check your heart rate from time to time. Most fitness facilities post a table of appropriate heart rates; keep your rate at the low end of the range appropriate for your age.

### Strength training

Building and maintaining muscle mass is an important part of any exercise program. But be cautious—avoid any weight training that involves holding your breath or straining. Get medical clearance before starting or continuing a weight training program.

---

### WHEN IS IT NOT SAFE TO EXERCISE?

*You should not exercise during this pregnancy if any of these conditions apply to you, until you have discussed your answers with your doctor.*

*Heart problems.*

*A serious lung condition and/or breathing problems.*

*High blood pressure.*

*Persistent vaginal bleeding during this pregnancy.*

*Low blood iron (anemia).*

*Carrying more than one baby.*

*Problems controlling (or my doctor is concerned about) my blood sugar.*

*My doctor has told me my baby is too small for its age in my uterus.*

*High risk for premature labour.*

*More information on exercise during pregnancy is available on the website of the Canadian Society for Exercise Physiology, at www.csep.ca*

## Do I exercise too much?

*If you check any of these boxes, you are overexerting yourself during your workout. It would be best to modify your exercise routine. If you have any questions, talk to your doctor.*

☐ I feel exhausted during
my workout.

☐ I feel very hot when I exercise.

☐ I am so short of breath that
I have trouble talking when
I exercise.

For more advice on exercising during pregnancy, call the Exercise and Pregnancy Hotline at 1-866-93-SPORT (77678). Run by the Women's College Ambulatory Care Centre and the Motherisk Program in Toronto, the hotline is a voicemail system that allows you to ask any questions you may have about exercise during pregnancy, and within 24 hours a sports medicine physician or trained athletic therapist will return your call. These professionals can help determine which exercises are safe for you.

## Rules to exercise by

### Aerobic exercise

Exercises using the large muscle groups include walking, swimming, stationary cycling, low-impact aerobics, cross-country skiing and aquafit.

Start slowly: take 15 minutes to warm up your muscles with gentle activity. Stretching or vigorous activity with "cold" muscles can give you unnecessary aches and pains or even injuries to muscles and ligaments.

Take rest breaks when you feel like it. Keep your heart rate at the low end of the target exercise heart rate for your age.

It is important to take 10 to 15 minutes to cool down, by working at less intensity until your heart rate returns to normal.

Drink plenty of water before, during, and after your exercise session.

Be careful when doing sports that require balance and coordination—your centre of gravity changes every day.

Avoid contact sports and activities that may cause you to fall or be hit, for example, downhill skiing, mountain climbing, floor hockey, water skiing, or soccer.

| Suggested heart rate target zones for aerobic exercise in pregnancy | | |
|---|---|---|
| Mother's age | Heart rate target | Beats per 10 seconds |
| Less than 20 years | 140 – 155 | 23 – 26 |
| 20 – 29 years | 135 – 150 | 22 – 25 |
| 30 – 39 years | 130 – 145 | 21 – 24 |
| More than 40 years | 125 – 140 | 20 – 23 |

*This applies to most healthy pregnant women. At the beginning of a new exercise or late in your pregnancy you should aim for the lower end of the heart rate target zone.*

### Strength training

Avoid any exercise that causes you to hold your breath and bear down at the same time, such as heavy weight-lifting routines.

Past the fourth month of pregnancy, abdominal exercises should be changed to use only the side-lying or standing positions.

You should avoid overstretching ligaments and tendons, which may be more flexible because of pregnancy hormones. Yoga and Pilates have not been studied in pregnancy, but qualified instructors will make adjustments in poses for safety if they know you are pregnant.

The most important muscles to tone now are the pelvic muscles. See page 46 for Kegel exercises.

### At the gym or fitness centre

Avoid exercises that strain your lower back, and always practice good posture.

Avoid exercising in a warm and humid environment. Hot tubs, saunas, and steam rooms, for example, should be avoided (or limited) to prevent an increase in your baby's body temperature.

PELVIC TILTS MAY HELP TO
RELIEVE YOUR BACKACHE

*This simple exercise done two or three times a day can help strengthen your abdominal muscles and take some pressure off your aching back. Relax your back. Exhale and pull your buttocks forward, pulling your pubic bone upward while keeping your lower back on the floor. Hold this position for a count of three and inhale and relax. Repeat five times.*

## Kegel exercises strengthen your pelvic floor muscles

Doing Kegel exercises is strength training for the muscles that surround your pelvic floor, getting them ready for the delivery. You can do Kegels anywhere and any time, but aim for 12 to 20 repetitions at least three times a day. It's easy to learn.

This will also help prevent urinary stress incontinence when you cough, lift, or laugh. Get used to the routine. It's a good habit for a lifetime. It helps you get back in shape after childbirth and helps prevent incontinence problems later in life.

1. Relax and sit or stand comfortably.

2. Find your pelvic muscle. Imagine that you are trying to hold back urine, or a bowel movement. Squeeze the muscles you would use to do that.

3. Tighten the muscles for five to 10 seconds.
   Do not hold your breath—breathe normally.
   Do not tighten your stomach or buttocks—keep them relaxed.

4. Now relax the muscles for about 10 seconds.

5. Repeat the cycle. Squeeze – hold – relax, 12 to 20 times.

## My pregnancy journal
## Notes from your prenatal visit at 10 to 16 weeks

This visit is scheduled for about four weeks after the first one. You will usually not have an extensive physical examination, but you will be weighed and have your blood pressure taken. The health care provider will check for the growth of the uterus and may also check your baby's heart rate.

At this visit, you and your health care provider will discuss the results of any tests that were ordered at the previous visit, and discuss any further testing or actions that may be required.

As with every prenatal visit, you should be well prepared and voice any concerns or questions you may want to discuss. Filling out this handbook can help prepare you for each visit. You will have notes from your last visit at your disposal, as well as a list of any questions that have occurred to you in the meantime.

If possible, it's a good idea for the expectant father to accompany you on your visit to the health care provider at least once. This will give him a chance to meet the person who is caring for his partner and voice any concerns or questions he may have. Other partners welcome to attend prenatal visits with you are a close friend, your mother, or another family member.

### My test results:

Hemoglobin: _____ (Normal 110-120 mg/L)
Blood type: _____
Immunity to:  German measles: Yes / No
            Chicken pox: Yes/No
Other results: _____
_____
_____
_____

MY DUE DATE:
_____

RECORDING MY PROGRESS

Date:
_____

Week of pregnancy:
_____

Blood pressure:
_____

Weight:
_____

Fetal heart rate:
_____

THINGS TO DISCUSS WITH MY
HEALTH CARE PROVIDER:

☐ Do I need genetic testing?

☐ Nausea and vomiting advice.

☐ How much weight should
I gain?

☐ Am I eating the right foods?

☐ Is it okay to have sex?

☐ Am I doing too much or too
little exercise?

☐ I have concerns about
family violence.

☐ What are Kegel exercises?

Other concerns:

# CHAPTER THREE

# Gentle growth:
## the second trimester

## HOW DOES THIS BABY MEASURE UP?

*The bone you can feel above your pubic area is the pubic bone. The top curve of your uterus is the fundus. Your health care provider may measure symphysis fundal height (SFH – the distance from your pubic bone to the top of your fundus) at each prenatal visit. This measurement is an indicator of the rate your baby is growing. The fundus usually reaches out of your pelvis by about the 12th week of pregnancy and reaches under your rib cage by the 36th week. Between the 18th and 30th week, the height of the fundus in centimetres is close to the age of the baby in weeks.*

*During this second trimester (15-25 weeks or 4 - 5 1/2 months), your pregnancy is considered well established and there is a much lower chance of having a miscarriage. You will probably feel more like your old self once you leave the morning sickness and minor discomforts of the first trimester behind you. Many women enjoy this part of their pregnancy because they are comfortable with their size and they like the way they look. Your baby will be growing at a rapid pace, and you will soon feel active movements from within your body as your baby rolls, somersaults, and kicks.*

## Your changing body

During your second trimester, the maturing placenta takes over most of the hormone production; your hormone levels will begin to even out, and you will probably feel more serene and settled.

You may worry if your friends or family comment that you seem small or large for your dates. But if you have been having regular prenatal visits, you know that your baby is growing at an acceptable rate. So why don't you look the right size?

Your body shape and size are related to many factors, not just the baby's size. Your pre-pregnancy height, weight and build, and whether or not this is your first pregnancy, are all factors. Short women tend to look bigger, and large boned or taller women tend to look smaller. Second-time mothers tend to have bigger bellies because the abdominal and uterine muscles have been stretched.

The pigmentation of your skin may have changed, so that you have a brownish vertical line down the middle of your abdomen, called the linea nigra. Some women develop brownish, uneven marks around the eyes and over the nose and cheeks. This condition usually disappears when hormone levels return to normal after your baby's birth.

As your breasts prepare themselves for feeding your baby, you may notice a little leaking of colostrum from the nipples. Colostrum is the clear sticky fluid your breasts prepare for baby's first feedings, before your breast milk comes in. It contains many important antibodies to protect your baby against infections.

In preparation for the birth, hormones cause the ligaments and cartilage of your pelvis and back to soften.

## Your developing baby

The baby really looks like a baby now; he's perfectly formed with all his body systems in place, functioning, and beginning to mature. The skin is red because the blood vessels are close to the surface. Some fat is starting to form under the skin, and a thick protective coating of a cheesy, whitish substance called vernix covers the entire body. The eyelids open and close by 26 weeks, the fingernails are full length and many babies have a visible hairline. Eyebrows and scalp hair become visible at the end of the 20th week and eyelashes can be seen at 24 weeks. The amniotic sac contains a large amount of fluid that is made up of nutrients for growth and the baby's urine. The umbilical cord is thick, strong, and very firm. This also helps prevent knots from forming.

## Preterm labour

Not everyone understands how important it is to carry a baby to full term. Some women hope for a premature baby, thinking a small baby may be easier to deliver.

In fact, premature labour is one of the most common problems in pregnancy and it is the cause of 75 percent of all newborn deaths in babies born without birth defects. Premature babies are more delicate and can have life-long problems related to their prematurity. In general, the more premature a baby is, the more severe the problems. Babies born before the 25th week usually do not survive without problems.

It is important to know early whether premature labour is occurring, as it sometimes can be stopped or delayed. This can provide time to give medicine that can help the baby, and to treat conditions causing premature labour.

### What causes premature labour?

Why some women develop premature labour, and others don't, is not well known. What we do know is that about half of all premature labours begin for unknown reasons to women whose pregnancies were otherwise normal. However, certain things seem to increase a woman's chances of going into early labour.

What you do during your pregnancy can help you carry your baby longer, and give him a better start. Research has shown that the more women know about the signs and risks of premature labour, the lower the rate of premature births.

In France, one long-term study showed a large reduction in overall prematurity rate when the following steps were taken:

- There was public education about preterm labour and the importance of healthy full term babies to society as a whole.
- Special seats on buses and special parking places were set aside for pregnant women.

---

**AM I AT RISK TO HAVE PREMATURE LABOUR**

*Check all the boxes that apply to you.*

- ☐ No regular prenatal care.
- ☐ High blood pressure.
- ☐ Great deal of stress in my life.
- ☐ Physical abuse from my partner or someone else.
- ☐ Carrying more than one fetus.
- ☐ A previous baby of mine was born too early.
- ☐ Body weight less than 45.5 kg (100 pounds).
- ☐ Chronic illness.
- ☐ A smoker.
- ☐ I quit smoking cigarettes, but not until after my 32nd week of pregnancy.
- ☐ Work long hours (more than 8 a day or shift work).
- ☐ My work is physically strenuous.

*If you checked one or more boxes, you are at risk to have premature labour and should talk to your doctor about precautions that may benefit you.*

- Pregnant women were encouraged to keep their own pregnancy record (much like this book).

**These are some of the risk factors for premature labour, and how the risk can be reduced:**

**Smoking**
It is best not to smoke during pregnancy. You can still benefit your baby if you quit smoking before you reach 32 weeks. Read the section on smoking on page 14.

**Working too hard**
Working long hours, doing strenuous kinds of work and being tired all the time can lead to a preterm birth. Read the section about "strenuous work" on page 58.

**Physical and emotional abuse**
When someone hurts you, they can also hurt your unborn baby. Even emotional abuse can lead to a preterm birth by significantly raising your stress levels. Please seek the help you need by calling a family crisis centre in your area.

**Incompetent cervix** – a rare condition in which the cervix dilates (opens) early and is associated with premature labour.

This can sometimes be diagnosed during a vaginal examination or by measuring the size of the cervix during an ultrasound. Sometimes this can be treated by sewing the cervix closed with a "drawstring" stitch and removing the sutures when the baby is full term.

**Fibroids in and/or on your uterus** can cause it to be misshapen. If fibroids large enough to deform the uterus are detected before pregnancy, they may be removed. Small fibroids usually don't cause problems during pregnancy.

*Premature labour can happen to anyone, but there are ways to help prevent it. Learn the signs of premature labour, and act right away if you think you are in labour.*

CALL THE HOSPITAL AND TALK TO A NURSE IN THE CASE ROOM:

*Phone:*

CALL YOUR DOCTOR:

*Phone:*

### Bleeding during second trimester

A small amount of bleeding can occur if the placenta begins to separate a bit from the lining of the uterus before labour starts. Each case of bleeding should be treated separately and may be treated differently depending on the cause. Always notify your health care provider about bleeding.

### Abdominal surgery during pregnancy

Sometimes abdominal surgery is needed when a woman is pregnant (for example, for appendicitis). Surgery that is wanted but not essential (elective) should be avoided until after the baby is born.

**Common infections in the mother** are vaginal, cervical, kidney or bladder infections.

You may have a bladder or kidney infection if you have pain when you urinate, if you have to go often, and when you do only a small amount of urine comes out. You may have an infection in your vagina or cervix if you notice an unusual vaginal discharge, have pain in your pelvis or groin area, or a fever. Notify your doctor.

### An underweight mother

Treatment depends on the cause of the problem. Sometimes this problem is helped by eating healthy, good food on a regular basis. Talk to your health care provider if you are underweight and having problems.

**Placenta previa** – a condition in which the placenta implanted and grew over the opening of the cervix (where the baby must come out). This can lead to hemorrhaging during labour.

This problem is usually found during routine ultrasound testing. The mother is often confined to bed for the last few weeks of pregnancy and the baby is usually delivered by caesarean section before labour has a chance to begin.

**Premature rupture of membranes** – the sac of amniotic fluid breaks or leaks before your baby reaches full term.

Some studies link this to infections in the uterus, but further research needs to be done. If your membranes rupture early, treatment depends on how much amniotic fluid is lost and how close to your due date you are. Notify your doctor, or health care provider.

**Gestational hypertension (high blood pressure caused by pregnancy)** – is treatable in various ways depending on the severity. Read more about this on page 67.

**Chronic illness in the mother.**
Some illnesses (diabetes, high blood pressure) may become out of control during the pregnancy, and in some situations the only way to stop the worsening condition is to deliver the baby. Sometimes the labour will begin too early on its own, and in other cases, the labour needs to be brought on (induced).

**WHEN TO CALL YOUR HEALTH CARE PROVIDER**

*Bleeding.*

*Leaking or a gush of fluid from your vagina.*

*Unexplained abdominal pain.*

*A decrease in the amount your baby moves inside you.*

*Your baby is not moving inside you.*

*Regular contractions of the uterus before your baby is due.*

*Unusual and constant headaches.*

*Blurred vision or spots before your eyes.*

*Dizziness.*

*Extreme tiredness.*

*Low dull backache.*

*If you are in a motor vehicle accident.*

*A feeling that something is not right.*

## How to feel and count contractions (tightenings)

1. *Lie down.*

2. *Using your fingertips, gently feel the entire surface of your lower abdomen.*

3. *When you notice a contraction (tightening or squeezing) over the surface of your uterus, time how long it lasts and how many minutes go by until it happens again.*

## What to do if you suspect you are in premature labour

1. *Stop whatever activity you are doing and rest.*

2. *Call your health care provider or labour ward at the hospital if you are not sure.*

3. *Go immediately to the nearest emergency room if:*
   - *your water breaks*
   - *you are bleeding*
   - *you are in pain*
   - *you are having regular contractions that are coming closer together and getting stronger.*

# Premature babies

About seven of every 100 babies will be born premature. They are born too early, before they reach full term. Normally, labour begins sometime after your 37th week of pregnancy and before the end of your 41st week. If labour starts before you reach your 37th week, your labour is considered early or premature.

The earlier a baby is born, the more problems he may face just to survive. The main reason these babies have problems is that their body organs are not ready to work all by themselves. These are called immature body systems. For example, a baby's lungs may not be fully able to take over the baby's breathing until close to the end of the pregnancy. Lungs that are not "ready" before the baby is born can result in mild to severe breathing problems for the newborn that may last a lifetime. An immature stomach and bowel can lead to feeding problems. When the immune system that protects your baby from catching certain diseases is not able to work on its own, your baby is more likely to get infections.

Premature babies can develop problems with their eyes and ears. They are redder and thinner than full term babies because the blood vessels are so close to the skin surface and they have very little fat under their skin. Without fat deposits, premature babies have problems staying warm. Under the abnormal circumstances of premature labour, they are also more likely to be delivered by caesarean section. As an expectant mother, it is by far in your best interest, and in the best interest of your unborn child, to do all that you can to prevent your child from being born before he reaches full term.

## Checking for premature labour

Labour begins when your uterus begins to contract at regular intervals. In addition, to prepare for the descent of your baby down the birth canal, the cervix will begin to thin out (efface) and open up (dilate). The protective mucous plug that formed at the entrance of your uterus during pregnancy may dislodge to produce a bloody mucous discharge called a show. Your waters may break; the sac filled with amniotic fluid that surrounds your baby may suddenly rupture.

The only way to know for sure if you are in premature labour is to be checked by a nurse/midwife or doctor to determine what the contractions are like and if the cervix is opening. At that time, the doctor, nurse or midwife will check your baby's heart rate and an ultrasound may be done to confirm the size, age, and position of your baby. Some hospitals have special tests to help determine if you are in premature labour.

If your labour has been confirmed as real labour (not false labour), and depending on how close to full term you are, you and your doctor will need to make a decision to try to stop your labour or to let the labour progress. Efforts to give your baby more time to mature inside your uterus are usually beneficial to your baby.

## What you can do to prevent premature labour

*There are other basic things which you can do in an effort to try to prevent your baby from being born too soon.*

**Quit smoking**
*Try to understand why you smoke, and seek help to learn other ways of dealing with these issues. Ask around in your community about "Quit Smoking" programs. Ask your doctor about programs to help you quit.*

**Eat properly**
*Talk to a registered dietitian about your eating habits. Plan your meals around the basic food groups and avoid junk food. Drink plenty of milk.*

**Get help if you need it**
*You have a right to feel safe. If you are being abused, call your local women's shelter and ask where you can go for help.*

**Get plenty of rest**
*Plan ahead to be sure a certain part of your day will be set aside for you to rest. Don't feel guilty for resting. It is very important during pregnancy.*

**Learn ways to reduce stress**
*Talk to people you trust about how you feel. Learn relaxation techniques such as meditation and self-massage to reduce your stress. Consider yoga.*

**Avoid strenuous work**
*Read what is considered strenuous work on page 58, and try hard not to do these things during pregnancy.*

**Avoid overexertion when exercising during pregnancy**
*Even though you are physically fit, it is important not to increase your work-out intensity during certain times of your pregnancy. Read more about this on pages 43-46.*

**Learn to recognize the signs of premature labour**
*Prenatal classes through your hospital or community are an excellent way to learn. Read about the signs of premature labour on page 52. Talk to your doctor.*

**Learn the steps to take if you think you are in premature labour**
*Talk to your doctor about what you should do. Write down the phone numbers to call and what your doctor wants you to do if you go into premature labour (see instructions on page 53).*

**Visit your doctor regularly during pregnancy**
*This is one of the most important things you can do to prevent premature labour because it gives your doctor a chance to find or prevent problems, which may cause your baby to be born early.*

## Is my work strenuous work?

*Check any of the following boxes that apply to your job.*

- ☐ *Stoop or bend over more than 10 times per hour.*
- ☐ *Climb a ladder more than three times in an eight-hour shift.*
- ☐ *Stand for more than four hours at one time.*
- ☐ *Climb stairs more than three times per shift.*
- ☐ *Work more than 40 hours per week.*
- ☐ *Work shift work.*
- ☐ *Will be expected to lift more than 23 kg (50 lbs) after the 20th week of my pregnancy.*
- ☐ *Will be expected to stand for more than four hours and lift more than 11 kg (24 lbs) after 24 weeks.*
- ☐ *Will be expected to stoop, bend or climb ladders after my 28th week.*
- ☐ *Will be expected to lift heavy items after my 30th week.*
- ☐ *Will be expected to stand still more than 30 minutes of every hour after 32 weeks.*

*If you checked any of the above boxes, the work may be considered too strenuous to do during your pregnancy. Your doctor may recommend that you change the work you do until after your baby is born. Read more about work during pregnancy on page 14.*

## Gestational diabetes

For some women, the pregnancy hormones change the way their bodies use insulin, and they go on to develop a type of diabetes because of the pregnancy. This is called gestational diabetes. Your health care provider may order a test for gestational diabetes around 24-28 weeks. Most will develop uncomplicated gestational diabetes, which means they will be able to control their blood sugar levels by eating a special diet and exercising. A small percentage may require insulin by injection to control their blood sugar levels. For most, the condition disappears after the baby is born, but some may go on to develop diabetes later in life. With preparation, good control, and professional care by a health care team, most women with gestational diabetes have a safe pregnancy and a healthy baby.

(For a discussion on the special requirements of women who have Type 1 or insulin-dependent diabetes at the time they become pregnant, see page 41).

## About fetal movement

A baby moves her arms and legs as a form of exercise and to move to a more comfortable position. If you are pregnant for the first time, you may not feel your baby move until you are in about your 19th week. If this is a second (or later) child, you will usually feel movement sooner, around the 17th week. From that point on, you should feel your baby move at different times of the day, every day. Keep in mind, a baby will have sleep periods throughout the day, and will have other times when she is more active. You may be asked to keep track of your baby's movements by counting the number of kicks you feel.

## About work

In normal, uncomplicated pregnancies, the type of work you do is not usually a problem. However, strenuous work or prolonged standing have been shown in some studies to be linked to a slight rise in such problems as low-birth-weight babies, premature labour, and miscarriage. To find out if your work is considered too strenuous, answer the questions in the sidebar on this page.

## Common discomforts in the second trimester

### Backaches
Your growing abdomen causes you to lean back to adjust your centre of gravity, which puts your back muscles under constant strain. In addition, the weight of the uterus in your pelvis, in combination with joint movement and softening, can also give you backaches during pregnancy. To prevent backaches, always try to sit up straight, avoid wearing high heels, lift using your leg muscles and not your back muscles (or resist lifting altogether), and avoid standing for long periods of time. Applying heat to your aching back or asking your partner for a back massage may help. Your doctor may suggest assessment or treatment by a licensed massage therapist, physiotherapist or chiropractor. Yoga, stretching, and relaxation techniques may prove beneficial and are worth investigating. Read about pelvic tilt exercises on page 46 that may help to relieve back strain. Be sure to change your body positions often and take time out of your busy day to lie down, put your feet up and relax.

### Constipation
During pregnancy, food movement through the bowel can become slower. This slowing-down process can lead to constipation. In addition, iron supplements can also cause constipation (and may turn your stools black). To help keep the stool from becoming dry and hardened, it is recommended that you drink at least eight glasses of fluid (juice, water, milk) daily. Getting regular exercise and eating plenty of fibre (ground flaxseed, whole grain bread, cereal products, psyllium), raw and dried fruits, and raw vegetables will help to move food through your intestine. If needed, your doctor may suggest a bulk forming agent or stool softener.

### Hemorrhoids
Many expectant mothers will develop hemorrhoids (varicose swollen or dilated veins of the rectum). Hemorrhoids often flare up during pregnancy because of the additional pressure your growing uterus places on the veins. If a woman strains to have a bowel movement because the stool is

---

**TIPS TO HELP REDUCE THE SWELLING IN YOUR LEGS AND FEET:**

Get regular exercise using your legs (swimming, walking).

Avoid crossing your legs.

Wear support hose and avoid socks with tight bands of elastic around the top.

Don't stand for long periods of time.

Raise your legs above the level of your heart whenever you can.

Drink 8 glasses of fluid each day.

Do not cut salt out of your diet.

hard, the hemorrhoids become worse, and may push out around the anal opening. Sometimes they are painful and bleed. Try to avoid constipation with a diet high in fibre, fruits, vegetables, and grains. Drink plenty of fluids to help keep your stool soft. Your doctor may suggest ointments to help shrink the hemorrhoids.

### Urinary tract infections (UTI)
The urinary tract involves the kidneys, ureters, bladder, and urethra. Infections in the urinary tract are common during pregnancy. Urine is made in the two kidneys. From each kidney, urine drips down tubes (ureters) into the bladder. When the bladder is full, urine exits the body through one tube called the urethra. Infections of this body system can sometimes be hard to detect. The common signs of an infection in your lower urinary tract (bladder) are: pain when you urinate, urinating unusually often, and only urinating a very small amount even though you felt a great urgency. This condition is easily treatable with antibiotics. An upper-urinary tract infection (involving the kidneys) is more serious. It can cause chills, fever, nausea, vomiting, backache, pain in the side, and lower abdominal discomfort. Women who are prone to urinary tract infections should be especially careful. UTIs are thought to be one of the causes of premature labour. Be sure to inform your doctor about flu-like symptoms during pregnancy because it may be something more serious.

### Indigestion and heartburn
If you feel a burning sensation at the back of your throat, lower in your food pipe (esophagus), or in your stomach, you may be suffering from indigestion related to pregnancy hormones and the pressure of a growing uterus.

It may help to eat small amounts of food more often, eating slowly and chewing your food well. You may also find it helps to drink fluids between meals, rather than during them. Avoid caffeine and greasy, spicy foods that are known to cause gas. Sit upright after a meal to allow time for the food to pass from the stomach into the intestine. Wear loose clothes. Only take antacids after speaking with your health care provider. Antacids can cause a rebound effect, in which your stomach produces even more acids after the effects of the antacid wear off, and antacids containing aluminum may interfere with absorption of certain minerals.

**Groin pain**
The round ligament that holds the uterus in place sometimes goes into spasms when it stretches as your baby grows. This stretching feels like a stabbing pain on one or both sides of your lower abdomen, or it can feel like a dull ache. These pains seem to be most common in the second trimester. Pregnant women sometimes worry these pains are premature labour pains. It may help to avoid turning your waist quickly. When you do feel pain, lean into it (bend toward the pain) to help relax the tension on the muscles. Lie down and get some rest. If the pain persists or becomes worse, and if changing positions does not relieve it, get checked either in the obstetrical ward of your hospital or your doctor's office.

**Dizziness if you lie flat on your back**
One of the largest blood vessels in your body, called the vena cava, transports blood from the lower part of your body back to your heart. It lies beside your spine. If your heavy uterus compresses the vena cava against your spine, the blood supply to your heart, lungs, and brain can be reduced. You may feel lightheaded and dizzy. This condition can also reduce your baby's blood supply. For this reason, it is important not to lie flat on your back during the last few months of pregnancy. Although lying on either side is fine, lying on your left side whenever possible is the best position to improve blood flow through the vena cava.

**Swelling of legs, ankles, and feet**
A small amount of swelling in your legs and ankles is normal during pregnancy. This type of swelling builds up each day and should all but disappear by the time you get up the next morning. It can be more of a problem if the weather is quite warm. Make sure you drink plenty of fluid (8 glasses/day) and do not cut out salt from your diet as your body requires some salt for day-to-day functions. Swelling of the hands or face may

mean you have a different, more serious problem. Read about high blood pressure on page 67.

### Stretch marks

For some women, reddish streaks, commonly referred to as stretch marks, develop over their breasts, abdomen, and thighs during pregnancy. To our knowledge, there has been no study done that says whether or not applying lotions and oils to your abdomen will reduce stretch marks. That being said, many women apply oil (particularly vitamin E oil or lanolin) to their abdomen. Whether or not this helps with stretch marks is unknown. Regardless, the rhythmic motion of rubbing your belly with lotions and oils will be relaxing for both you and your unborn child and it certainly can't do any harm.

### Dry, itchy skin

Avoid the use of soaps (if you must use soap, try glycerine soap) because they tend to wash away the natural lubricants in your skin. Lying in a tub of water for too long can also dry out your skin by washing away natural oils. Putting oil or an oatmeal-based softener in the bath will help. If you use bath oil, take care getting out of the tub, which may become slippery. After a bath or shower, apply body lotion to damp skin to help keep your skin supple, soft, and moisturized.

# My pregnancy journal
## 16 to 24 weeks

As at the last visit, your examination will include weighing and measuring you and your baby.

At about 16 to 18 weeks, your doctor may suggest a screening ultrasound test. This test will enable your doctor to measure the size of your baby, helping to reconfirm your baby's due date.

*Date:*

*Week of pregnancy:*

*Blood pressure:*

*Weight:*

*Fetal heart rate:*

**My test results:**

Gestational diabetes test:          (Normal = 3.8-7.8 mmol/L)

Ultrasound results:

THINGS TO DISCUSS WITH MY
HEALTH CARE PROVIDER:

☐ *Am I at risk for
premature labour?*

☐ *Is my work too strenuous?*

*Other concerns:*

# Home stretch: the third trimester

Date:

Week of pregnancy:

Blood pressure:

Weight:

Fetal heart rate:

*As you near the end of your pregnancy, you will probably begin to feel a bit anxious and tired, and will be looking forward to having the baby. During your last month of pregnancy, your prenatal visits will be more frequent, as often as once every week for the last month. Your blood pressure, urine, and the position of the baby will be checked at each visit.*

*Most women go into labour some time after their 38th week and before the end of their 41st week of pregnancy.*

## Your changing body

During your third trimester, you are visibly pregnant. The top of the uterus will grow from above the navel to under the rib cage and your abdomen will increasingly protrude. You may feel increasing discomfort from this, feeling pressure on your ribs, stretching of the abdominal muscles, and pressure in the pelvis. You may feel sharp pains in the groin or vagina, as your baby's head goes into the pelvis.

## Your developing baby

Your baby is fully formed and growing steadily from 25-26 weeks, when his weight will be 700-900 grams (1 1/2 to 2 pounds). By 35-36 weeks, he will weigh 2500 grams (5 1/2 pounds). By the time he is ready to be born, he will weigh between 3000 and 4000 grams (6 1/2 to 9 pounds).

Although all the organ systems are there, they are still growing and maturing. The baby's arms and legs are bent close to his body. He has periods of activity and rest (like a newborn does).

Breathing movements become regular at 20-21 weeks. Your baby's lungs become capable of breathing air at between 26-29 weeks. The baby is beginning to feel crowded inside the uterus, but you should still feel active movement every day.

A good volume of amniotic fluid surrounds and protects him.

## High Blood Pressure

Hypertension is the medical term for high blood pressure. Expectant mothers who develop high blood pressure because they are pregnant are said to have the condition known as gestational hypertension. This condition is also known as toxemia or as pre-eclampsia.

When a woman has gestational hypertension, her blood vessels constrict, which may reduce the blood supply to her placenta. This, in turn, may reduce the blood supply to her baby and slow the baby's growth. In addition to the high blood pressure, this condition often causes excess protein to spill over into the urine, and swelling of the face, hands, feet, and ankles. Read about normal swelling on page 61.

### Who will develop it?
About seven of every 100 expectant mothers will develop gestational hypertension. Most will be first-time mothers. Women who had high blood pressure before getting pregnant are also more likely to develop the condition.

### AM I AT RISK OF GETTING GESTATIONAL HYPERTENSION?

*Check the boxes that apply to you.*

☐ My first pregnancy.

☐ High blood pressure before I got pregnant.

☐ Have diabetes.

☐ Have medical condition which causes my kidneys not to work properly.

☐ Carrying more than one baby.

☐ Very low income.

☐ Younger than 18.

☐ Older than 35.

*If you checked any boxes, you are at risk of developing gestational hypertension.*

### SIGNS OF HIGH BLOOD PRESSURE

*If you have any of these symptoms, call your doctor right away.*

• Pain in the upper right part of the abdomen.

• Constant, severe, or changing headaches.

• Spots in front of your eyes and/or blurred vision.

• Unusual swelling, particularly around the face, and weight gains that are sudden and more than one pound per day.

▶ YOUR DOCTOR WILL CHECK
FOR HIGH BLOOD PRESSURE
(GREATER THAN 140/90)
AND PROTEIN IN YOUR URINE.

**Treatment for high blood pressure in pregnancy**
If you are diagnosed with gestational hypertension, every attempt will be made by your health care team to allow your baby to remain in the uterus for as long as possible provided this doesn't cause an increased risk to you or your baby.

In a mild form of the condition, bed rest is usually enough to bring down the slightly high blood pressure. When resting, you will be asked to lie on your sides (never on your back) to improve the blood supply to your uterus and kidneys. In some situations, your doctor may recommend that you be hospitalized until your blood pressure is under control, and/or you may be given medication to help lower your blood pressure.

Severe gestational hypertension results in extremely high blood pressure and can cause problems in the mother's kidneys, liver, and brain. Problems in the brain may cause seizures. Untreated and severe gestational hypertension can lead to the death of the mother and her baby, although this is very rare today. Drugs will be given in an attempt to lower the mother's blood pressure and to prevent seizures. When this condition is severe, the best thing to do is to deliver the baby.

## Feeding your baby

Over the past 20 years, breastfeeding has been studied a great deal. Researchers have identified many clear benefits for both the mother and the child. Based on this scientific evidence, the Society of Obstetricians and Gynaecologists of Canada (SOGC), the Canadian Paediatric Society, the World Health Organization (WHO), and the United Nation's Children's Fund (UNICEF) agree that the best food source for the first six months of life is breast milk.

## Why breast is best

Women have always breastfed their children and breastfeeding is still the ideal way to feed children. Today, 85 percent of Canadian women having babies will breastfeed. As a nursing mother, you will receive emotional and practical support from many sources.

Breast milk, including the colostrum, contains antibodies that boost your baby's immune system and help fight disease. This stronger immune system lowers the chance of your baby getting an infection. A few examples of infections are colds, ear infections, stomach flus, baby measles, kidney infections, pneumonia, and meningitis. Breastfed babies have a lower chance of contracting some bowel disorders (e.g., celiac disease, Crohn's disease), asthma, allergies, and eczema. Breast milk even lowers the chances of appendicitis. Breast milk is more easily absorbed and quicker to digest than formula, so breastfed babies tend to have fewer problems with constipation and stomach upset. Babies are hardly ever allergic to breast milk, but can have mild to severe allergic reactions to formula.

Breast milk contains omega-3 fatty acids, which are very important for brain development. Breast milk also has hormonally active proteins that are important in the development of your baby's gut, nerves, and disease-fighting cells.

Breastfeeding is also great for you. Breastfeeding triggers the release of certain hormones that will help your uterus return to its normal size.

---

### BREASTFEEDING—GETTING STARTED WITH COLOSTRUM

*Most babies are ready to nurse within the first hour. Until your white milk comes in (usually 2–4 days after the birth), your breasts will produce a yellow, milk-like substance called colostrum. This colostrum contains antibodies, omega-3 fatty acids, and the perfect balance of nutrients, minerals, vitamins, and trace elements for your baby. Your baby will be born with extra water stores and fat to use until your white milk comes in. In the meantime, the colostrum feedings are perfect for baby and all she needs. Most babies lose weight after birth because they use up these fat and water stores. This weight loss should not be more than seven percent of their birth weight. It is best to breastfeed your newborn whenever he or she seems hungry. Babies should not receive water supplements.*

Breastfeeding also helps to protect you from breast, ovarian, and uterine cancer. Breastfeeding encourages closeness and a special bond between you and your baby. Finally, breastfeeding is free and involves no preparation. Formula feeding will cost $1500 or more during the first year.

If you are considering bottle-feeding, learn as much as you can about both methods. Consider your feelings, your partner's feelings, your cultural beliefs, nutrition, and cost.

Talk to other women and to such organizations as the La Leche League Canada Breastfeeding Referral Service (1-800-665-4324) or your local public health nurse for more information. In some areas, breastfeeding clinics and private breastfeeding experts, called lactation consultants, are also available to help you.

If you do decide not to breastfeed, your health care providers will respect your decision and support you.

## Breastfeeding: myths and facts

1. *Breastfeeding is easy, natural, and instinctual.*

   *Yes, once you and your baby have caught on and developed your own routine, breastfeeding may be easy, natural and instinctual. But until then, it may involve lots of trial and error and can be frustrating. Don't be afraid to ask for help. Stick with it–it's worth it.*

2. *I shouldn't start breastfeeding because I'm not sure I can continue for more than two or three months.*

   *If in doubt, start. It is worthwhile for your baby to be nursed for any period of time, even just a few days. This way, the baby will get the advantages of your milk and it keeps your options open.*

3. *Nursing mothers are tied to their babies.*

   *Nursing or otherwise, your newborn baby will need frequent feedings and care. Yes, nursing requires mothers to remain close to their babies, but this is not necessarily a bad good thing.  You may find benefit in knowing that you are always there to breastfeed and comfort your baby, and unlike formula, breastfeeding requires no preparation time. In the early months, take the baby with you and you will likely find breastfeeding can be both convenient and flexible.*

4. *Every woman can produce enough milk to feed her baby.*

   *Usually this is true, but some mothers may not have enough milk and will need to supplement.  Remember that nursing your baby stimulates your body's milk supply to meet your baby's exact demands.*

5. *Babies must suck differently from a bottle than from a breast.*

   *True. Bottle feeding requires a different type of sucking than breastfeeding, so the baby may become confused at the difference between your nipple and the nipple of a bottle.*

6. *If I breastfeed, my breasts will be more likely to sag afterward.*

   *Your breasts may look a bit different after breastfeeding, but most changes in breast tissue (such as sagging) happen over time and are due to the aging process.*

7. *If I breastfeed, I shouldn't bottle feed at all.*

   *For success at breastfeeding, it is best to avoid introducing a bottle at first to prevent nipple confusion.  Once your milk supply and the baby's technique are well established (at least six weeks), bottle feeding can be introduced – ideally with expressed breast milk.*

8. *Children should be weaned at six months of age.*

   *Not true. Breast milk is the best milk for babies and toddlers. The World Health Organization (WHO) recommends breastfeeding for two years or more. If breastfeeding is working well for you, there is no reason to quit before your child does so on his or her own.*

9. *Some mothers should not breastfeed.*

   *Very rarely, women have to take medication that can harm the baby through breastfeeding.  Women who are HIV-positive or who are abusing street drugs or alcohol should not breastfeed.*

10. *Women with breast implants cannot breastfeed.*

    *Many women with implants can breastfeed.*

11. *Blue or watery milk has no nutritional value.*

    *Not true. Foremilk, almost clear and bluish in colour, is rich in protein, vitamins and minerals. Hind milk, white in color, is rich in fat.*

12. *The small amount of colostrum is enough for your baby in the first few days.*

    *This is true. Colostrum provides both water and sugar, as well as protein, minerals and important antibodies (protection from disease) that your baby cannot obtain elsewhere.*

13. *Breastfed babies should be given a soother (pacifier) to help them learn to suck.*

    *Not recommended. Pacifiers may teach your baby poor sucking technique, hide his or her hunger signs, and are one way that disease is spread.*

14. *It is best to breastfeed a baby whenever he or she seems hungry.*

    *True. Breastfeeding your baby on demand makes for a more satisfied baby and successful breastfeeding. In the beginning, babies usually nurse 8-12 times each day.*

15. *Both breastfed and bottle-fed babies need water supplements.*

    *Not true. Breast milk contains enough water to meet your baby's needs. Water has no nutritional value, and feeding your baby water by bottle can lead to a reduced appetite at feeding time.*

16. *If I am going to breastfeed, I will have to be very careful to eat properly.*

    *It is always wise to practice good nutrition. However, unless you are on an extreme diet, your milk will be of an excellent quality.*

17. *I have to wean before I go back to work.*

    *Not true. Mothers who return to work have a number of choices. Some mothers nurse when they are at home and express or pump their milk while at work, for the baby to have the next day. Other mothers nurse when they are home and use frozen breast milk or formula when they are away.*

## Group B Streptococcus (GBS)

At about 36 weeks, you will likely be tested for the presence of the group B Streptococcus (GBS) bacteria. These are different from the bacteria that cause strep throat. If these bacteria are in your body but you don't have any signs of infection, you are said to be colonized (positive). The GBS bacteria are usually found in your vagina or rectum and can infect your bladder, kidneys, or uterus. Infections from GBS are usually not serious for the mother and are readily treated with antibiotics. However, if these bacteria are passed on to your baby during childbirth, there is a remote chance your baby could become infected, too. Babies who are infected with GBS may have mild to severe problems that may affect their blood, brain, lungs, and spinal cord.

### Testing for group B Streptococcus

The most common way to test a woman for the presence of GBS bacteria is to swab her vagina and rectum with a Q-tip, which is then placed in special solution to see if the bacteria grow. This is called doing a "culture." Sometimes your doctor may also look for the presence of bacteria in your urine.

### Treatment for group B Streptococcus (GBS)

No method of testing and treating mothers infected with GBS prevents all cases of the GBS bacteria from being passed on to babies. It is very rare, but babies still die of GBS infection.

If at 36 weeks you test positive for GBS, you will be offered antibiotics during labour. If you have not been tested yet for GBS, then you may be treated with antibiotics in labour if you are thought to be at higher risk (see sidebar).

## What to expect in hospital

Obstetrical health care in Canada has changed since your mother gave birth to you, and even more since her mother was "confined," as childbirth was once called.

---

**YOU MAY BE AT HIGHER RISK TO PASS GBS ON TO YOUR BABY IF YOU:**

1. Start labour before you reach 37 weeks.

2. Reach full term, but your membranes have been ruptured more than 18 hours before your expected time of delivery.

3. Have an unexplained, mild fever.

4. Have already had a baby who had a GBS infection.

5. Have (or had) a bladder or kidney infection that was caused by the GBS bacteria.

CHILDBIRTH IS A NORMAL LIFE EXPERIENCE, NOT AN ILLNESS.

## FAMILY-CENTERED CARE HOSPITAL CHECKLIST

*My hospital:*

☐ *will accept the birthing plan I have developed, or has a standard birthing plan I can adapt to suit my needs.*

☐ *will encourage me to have a labour coach.*

☐ *offers the support of a professional labour support person.*

☐ *encourages skin-to-skin contact (kangaroo care) immediately after birth.*

☐ *encourages breastfeeding, starting right after the birth.*

☐ *will not separate my baby and me unless it is medically necessary.*

☐ *allows my baby to stay in my room with me and my family.*

☐ *treats birth as a normal and natural process, not an illness.*

☐ *will try to assign only one nurse to me during my labour and delivery. (Some hospitals may not have enough staff to do this, but most will try).*

☐ *accepts my individual religious beliefs, and wants to do all they can to accommodate my cultural needs.*

☐ *allows me the freedom with regard to procedures, labour positions, delivery positions, and pain control.*

☐ *has flexible visiting hours for close family members.*

Over the past 20 years or so, physicians, nurses, and mothers have promoted changes in the approach of obstetrical care. Family-centered maternity care has replaced the strict medical approach to care. Routine hospital practices were studied to be sure they were beneficial to women and some standard procedures such as enema and episiotomy were dropped from routine care.

Hospital obstetrical units have adapted to meet women's needs, by becoming warm and homelike places to have a baby, while offering excellent medical care when it is needed.

Care has been individualized, with women being encouraged to prepare a birthing plan reflecting their desires and options.

Birthing units and LDRP (labour, delivery, recovery and postpartum) units were opened throughout Canada with help and guidance from obstetricians, family physicians, midwives and nurses.

To improve the safety of childbirth for the mother, and to make the event more enjoyable, most hospitals in Canada now promote the family-centered approach to maternity (obstetrical) care. When hospital maternity care programs include every member of the family, stronger and healthier families appear. Fathers and family tend to be more supportive when they feel needed and included in the childbirth process. Although it is usually best not to have young children present during labour and childbirth, it is recommended that they join their family as soon after the birth as possible to welcome the new family member.

*If you checked most of these boxes, your hospital offers a family-centered approach to maternity care. If not, then most health care workers will still try very hard to meet your needs. You may find that by giving the staff your completed birthing plan, you may still be able to achieve the birth you desire.*

### The obstetrical nurse/midwife

The current trend in caring for normal pregnancies is to recognize the importance of the people who offer human support and understanding for the labouring woman. Many studies show that when an experienced obstetrical nurse or midwife closely helps a labouring woman, the risk of problems for the mother and the baby is less. Ideally, your labour and delivery nurse will also take care of you and your baby after the birth. Studies have shown you are more likely to have a normal labour and birth if you have a support person with you.  Besides nurses and midwives, important labour support can come from your partner, other family members, friends, or a professional doula.

### Rooming in

In family-centered care, most babies "room in," staying in their mothers' hospital rooms and not in the newborn nursery. Under normal circumstances, it is healthy and best for mothers and their newborns to stay together in the same room from birth to discharge. In the past, the newborn nursery was considered cleaner, and therefore safer for your baby than staying in the room with you.  In reality, the opposite is true. When an infant stays in the same room as the mother, the mother does most of the handling. In the nursery, many different nurses, all of whom may be handling other infants, handle the infant. In spite of all the hand washing nurses do, the risk of infection for a newborn is greater in the nursery.

## Writing your birthing plan

A birthing plan is a written document that tells your doctor and the hospital staff what kind of childbirth you would like and how you would like your baby cared for after he is born.

### How to write a birthing plan

A birthing plan should be simple and less than one page long. Try to be realistic in your requests and keep in mind that your childbirth experience will include your health care team, yourself, your partner, the baby, and your family. Your birth plan will be most effective if you write down what

BIRTHING PLAN

*Try not to be too detailed or complicated. No one can predict how your labour and birth will progress, so it is important that your birthing plan be flexible.*

you want to happen and your preferences if what you want to happen isn't going to happen. For example, you may write, "I would prefer not to have an IV in place throughout labour, but only if and when it is needed."

**When to write a birthing plan**
Usually, a birthing plan is written after you talk over your childbirth plans with your doctor and once you know what your hospital offers in terms of routines and care. It is also a good idea to talk it over with your partner and your family if they are going to be involved in some way. However, it is your body, and your family needs to understand that you are the only one who can make some of the more personal decisions (for example, about pain control). Make two copies and give one to your doctor and one to the hospital staff before the end of your eighth month or as you enter the hospital in early labour.

Many hospitals now have a draft birth plan for you to use as a template. You can also use the example provided by the Society of Obstetricians and Gynaecologists of Canada in their Healthy Beginnings Clinical Practice Guidelines found on their website: www.sogc.org

*The following websites provide further information on umbilical cord blood banking:*

- *The Society of Obstetricians and Gynaecologists of Canada: www.sogc.org*

- *Canadian Cord Blood Registry: www.ccbr.ca*

- *The Alberta Cord Blood Bank: www.acbb.ca*

- *Hema-Quebec: www.hema-quebec.qc.ca*

## Umbilical cord blood banking

After your baby is born and the umbilical cord is cut, there is a length of umbilical cord still attached to the placenta. This cord is filled with a small amount of blood, some of which is routinely tested for the baby's blood type and blood oxygen and pH levels. The remainder of the blood, along with the placenta once it is expelled, is discarded as medical waste.

The blood in the umbilical cord contains special cells called stem cells which can be used to treat children with cancers or other bone marrow diseases such as leukemia or lymphoma. In other words, these cells could save someone's life. You can choose to donate the umbilical cord blood. At present in Canada, there are two public umbilical cord banks that store blood for the public good.

## Things to think about in your birthing plan

We have listed some of the common things women talk about in their birthing plans. You don't have to mention all of them in your own birthing plan. If something is not as important to you, you can leave it out. If you think of something else that is not on this list, feel free to include it in your birthing plan.

**The labour coach**
Studies show that when a labouring woman is continuously supported by someone who cares for her (a labour coach), she will have a more positive experience. The hospital will provide you with a professional labour support partner (maternity nurse) who will help you during labour, delivery, and after the baby is born.

**Enema**
Health care providers do not routinely give enemas. However, some women find that having an enema relieves pressure in the lower bowel, particularly if they were constipated before labour.

**Shave preps**
Most hospitals today do not routinely shave the pubic area.

**Intravenous line (IV)**
Unless your pregnancy is considered a high-risk pregnancy, or unless there is a medical reason, most hospitals do not start routine IVs. An IV provides access to your blood stream quickly in case of an emergency. Sometimes an IV is the best way to give you certain medications, such as antibiotics, labour-starting drugs, or as required for an epidural. Some women benefit from the extra IV fluids if they become dehydrated during labour or if they wish to have an epidural.

**Blood tests**
Usually routine blood tests are not done if a pregnancy is considered low risk and normal. Sometimes, certain blood tests are needed (for example "blood sugar tests" if you are a diabetic) to make sure everything is going along well.

**Inducing labour**
If your labour has not started by the end of your 41st week, or if there are other medical complications, your doctor may consider inducing labour. Labour should not be induced without good reason. Read the section about overdue babies on page 88.

**Monitoring the fetus**
Evidence shows that during normal labour it is best to monitor the baby at regular intervals using methods that do not limit your movements. Under special circumstances, it will be necessary to monitor the baby using continuous fetal monitors (see page 96).

**Movement during labour**
Most hospitals today encourage mothers to move about freely during the early stages of labour. Evidence shows that this mild form of exercise in the early stages of labour helps labour to move along more quickly.

**Eating and drinking during labour**
In the very early stages of labour, eating and drinking small amounts may prevent dehydration and help keep your strength up. However, when you are in active labour, most women do not feel like eating, but may wish to have small amounts of clear fluids. In some high-risk circumstances, food and drink may be restricted.

**Pain relief**
There are many different ways to help you cope with the pain of labour and childbirth, ranging from special breathing to an epidural block. When a labouring mother's pain is under control, she is better able to help with

the birth. It is okay to choose natural childbirth (no pain killers) but it is also okay to change your mind if the pain becomes unbearable. Read more about ways to make labour easier in Chapter Six.

## Pushing

At the end of active labour, the urge to push your baby out is strong; suddenly you will want to bear down (push). The body naturally wants to bear down a few short times during each contraction, and take breaths in and out between pushes. Evidence shows this method gives the baby the most oxygen. Sometimes a different method is encouraged in hospitals. Mothers may be encouraged to take a deep breath and hold it, then push one hard, long push with a deep breath at the end. Evidence shows this method may lower the baby's oxygen levels over time, but may speed up the delivery. Sometimes, the cervix is not quite ready for the baby to move through, and you may be instructed not to push. If that happens, you will be told what you can do to avoid pushing (such as a knee-to-chest position or special breathing).

## Delivery positions

There is clear evidence today that sitting upright or semi-sitting for delivery is best. These positions seem to lower the time it takes to push a baby out. Lying on your side is also a natural delivery position which has many benefits. Squatting down can be beneficial because it improves the angle of the pelvis, to give the baby more room to come out, and the force of gravity enables the baby to slide out more quickly. Today, women's legs are no longer strapped into stirrups.

## Episiotomy

There is no evidence to support routine episiotomy (making an incision or cut to widen the vaginal opening). There are more benefits to avoiding episiotomies, such as less pain after the baby is born, better sexual function later, and less relaxation of the pelvic muscles. Sometimes, an episiotomy is necessary to relieve pressure or to deliver a baby in distress more quickly.

### Cutting the umbilical cord

A slight delay in cutting the umbilical cord of about 30 seconds may be of benefit to your baby, as it can improve blood supply. This may be especially beneficial for premature babies. If the baby's father wishes to cut the cord, this can also be arranged.

### Skin-to-skin contact

Studies have shown that cuddling and skin-to-skin contact with your baby immediately after birth, known as kangaroo care, is important to your baby's adjustment to life outside of the womb.

### Religious or cultural beliefs

Feel free to list your needs in this area, for example, traditions, beliefs, and expectations for yourself, the baby, and your family.

### Rooming in

Studies show it is best for you and your baby to stay and sleep in the same room together. Babies who room in are handled mostly by their mothers. Babies in the nursery are handled by many people. Therefore, the risk of infection for a baby is greater in the nursery. Rooming in is a good opportunity for you and your baby to bond with each other.

### Caesarean birth

If you know you are having a caesarean section, you may want to think about what kind of pain relief you want, or if you want your partner to attend. If you were to be faced with an emergency delivery, what would your choices be?

# Breastfeeding

### Starting to breastfeed
Evidence shows the best time to begin breastfeeding is within 30-60 minutes after birth, when the baby is most alert. This is also the perfect time to begin bonding with your baby and to have skin-to-skin contact.

### Feeding schedules
Studies show it is best to breastfeed your baby whenever your baby seems hungry and not on a regular schedule. This is called demand feeding.

### Just milk
Studies show that most breastfed babies do not need feedings of anything other than breast milk. Water feedings using a bottle tend to lessen the baby's appetite, and the two different nipples may confuse the baby.

### Asking for help
There are many ways that you can find help for breastfeeding. Sometimes the help will be offered, and sometimes you may have to ask for it. In many areas there are home nursing programs, public health clinics, breastfeeding clinics, and professional lactation (breastfeeding) consultants.

RECORDING MY PROGRESS

Date:

Week of pregnancy:

Blood pressure:

Weight:

Fetal heart rate:


THINGS TO DISCUSS WITH MY
HEALTH CARE PROVIDER:

• Am I at risk for premature labour?





• Is my work too strenuous?

# My pregnancy journal
## 24 to 32 weeks

Your examination will include weighing and measuring you and your baby. As at your last visit, signs of premature labour will be discussed, as well as how you are getting along with minimizing the risks. Are you continuing to eat well and get regular exercise? Are you protecting your baby from cigarette smoke and alcohol? Are the conditions at work stressful or physically tiring? Do you get enough rest?

If you have had any tests or a screening ultrasound since your last office visit, the results will be reviewed with you.

As at other visits, your plans for the big day and what you can expect will be reviewed. These discussions and your reading will help you get a clear picture of the choice you have for birthing your baby, and you will begin to develop opinions about what you think is best for you, your baby, your partner, and your family.

## My pregnancy journal

### 32 to 36 weeks

You will have prenatal visits every 2-3 weeks now. Your examinations will include weighing and measuring you and your baby. As at your last visits, your doctor will be looking for any signs of premature labour. Your baby and how she is growing will receive a lot of the attention.

You and your doctor will review your birthing plan (pages 75-80) at this visit and talk about any concerns you may have about childbirth.

Eating well is still an important concern as your baby is growing rapidly.

RECORDING MY PROGRESS

Date:

Week of pregnancy:

Blood pressure:

Weight:

Fetal heart rate:

THINGS TO DISCUSS WITH MY HEALTH CARE PROVIDER:

Questions about breastfeeding:

Questions about my birth plan:

Weight gain/nutrition:

Other concerns:

_____
_____
_____
_____
_____
_____
_____
_____
_____
_____
_____
_____
_____
_____
_____
_____
_____
_____
_____
_____
_____
_____
_____
_____
_____
_____
_____
_____
_____
_____
_____
_____
_____
_____
_____
_____

CHAPTER FIVE

# All ready to go

*How are you getting to the hospital?*
*Is your car reliable?*
*Make a back-up plan.*

*How easily will you be able to reach*
*your labour support partner when*
*you go into labour?*

*How far from the hospital are you?*
*It is best to drive the distance and*
*time it. Consider the road conditions*
*and rush hour traffic possibilities*
*when you do. Plan an alternative*
*route in case of road obstructions.*

*Where are you suppose*
*to park the car?*

*Do you need to pre-register at the*
*hospital or can you just show up?*

*Who will take care*
*of your children at home?*

*Do you need someone to feed*
*your pets for you while you are*
*hospitalized?*

## Your changing body

Some time toward the end of pregnancy, most babies will settle into the head down, or the engaged, position. Some people also call this event the time when the baby "drops" or "lightening." It can be normal if this doesn't occur until just before labour starts. When your baby settles deep into your pelvis, the head will rest on top of your cervix. You will feel different and look as though you are carrying the baby much lower. The good news is that after the baby drops, some of the pressure on your ribs will be relieved and you will probably breathe a little more easily. Sometimes, however, this low and heavy weight can add to muscle strain and backaches.

The uterus is starting to have "practice contractions" (Braxton Hicks contractions) that may or may not be painless and should be irregular. You may notice them, or you may not. Because of the pressure the uterus places on the blood vessels in your pelvis, the swelling in your feet and ankles may be more noticeable. But swelling of the face and hands may be a sign of a more serious problem. (Read about gestational hypertension on page 67).

Your pelvic bones have loosened and may ache, especially at the back. You may notice your breasts leaking some colostrum, leaving a crusty film on your nipples (although many women do not produce colostrum before the baby is born). Your breasts may feel full and heavy and will need a good support bra for the months to come, particularly when you breastfeed. Your abdomen may become so stretched that your navel pushes out. The brown pigment of your skin can become very noticeable near the end of pregnancy.

## Your developing baby at full term

A baby at full term is plump and rounded. She will measure 46-51 cm (18-20 inches) in length, and weigh between 3000 and 4000 grams (6 1/2 to 9 pounds.) Most of the cheesy vernix that protected the skin is gone now, and the bit that remains is slippery and will help during the birth process.

The baby's eyes are open when awake, and closed when sleeping. Her lungs are now producing surfactant that will help them prepare for the first breath. A full-term baby's immune system is still not mature. To counter-balance this problem, your baby will get antibodies from you, via your placenta before she is born and more from your breast milk (colostrum) after she is born. The placenta is now about 20 cm (8-10 inches) in diameter and about 2.5 cm (1 inch) thick.

## Common discomforts in late pregnancy

### Leg, calf, and foot cramps
Many women experience cramps during the last three months of pregnancy, mostly at night. These sudden cramps in the thighs, legs, calves, or feet can be very painful and are usually followed by an ache that lasts for a long time. When a cramp strikes, try this: in spite of the pain, point your toe toward your knee in an effort to stretch the muscle straight again. Then keep your foot in this flexed position while you slowly and carefully make circling movements with your lower leg. Afterward, deeply massage the cramped muscle to improve the blood supply to that area.

### Difficulty sleeping
Sleeping problems are common throughout pregnancy, and most common in the last trimester. Your large abdomen makes finding a comfortable position a challenge, and the added trips to the bathroom at night don't help either. Try using a number of large pillows to prop up your legs, abdomen, and back (but do not lie flat on your back). Ask your partner for a back massage to help you drift off to sleep. It may help to take a warm bath before going to bed. Try keeping the bedroom temperature cool. Avoid sleeping pills; they can cross through the placenta and make your baby sleepy.

---

### PACKING YOUR SUIT

*It is best to pack your suitc[ase] weeks before your due date[...] the baby arrives early. Onc[e] labour begins, you may not have time to remember everything you want to bring.*

*A helpful checklist for you:*

- ☑ *This book, pen, paper*
- ☐ *Copy of your birthing plan*
- ☐ *Housecoat, nightgown, and slippers*
- ☐ *Loose-fitting clothes to go home in*
- ☑ *Extra pair of socks*
- ☑ *Bra (nursing or good support bra)*
- ☑ *Underwear*
- ☑ *Sanitary napkins*
- ☑ *Toothbrush, toothpaste*
- ☑ *Hairbrush, comb*
- ☐ *Camera, batteries, film*
- ☐ *Change for phones and vending machines*
- ☐ *Labour support items such as massage oil for back rubs*
- ☑ plastic bag for soiled clothing

*A helpful checklist for your baby:*

- ☑ *Clothes to go home in*
- ☑ *Diaper(s)*
- ☑ *Receiving blanket*
- ☑ *Warmer blanket*
- ☑ *Hat,* socks
- ☐ *Car seat*

TRUE LABOUR VS. FALSE LABOUR

*If you are in doubt as to whether your labour is true or false, it may be helpful to time the contractions. Write down how many minutes apart they are, from the start of one contraction until the start of the next, and note how long each one lasts. If possible, keep a record for one hour.*

1. STRENGTH OF CONTRACTIONS

TRUE
*The contractions will get steadily stronger and you will be able to feel your uterus hardening.*

FALSE
*The contractions do not get progressively stronger.*
*They may weaken at times and even disappear for a while.*

## Vaginal discharge

The discharge from your vagina normally increases during pregnancy, and it can become even more plentiful (even messy at times) during your last trimester. Wearing a sanitary mini pad may make you feel more comfortable and protected. This discharge should look and feel like the white of a raw egg. It should not be bloody (unless it is your mucous plug), watery (this could be amniotic fluid), or foul smelling (this may mean you have an infection). You should not have any pain, itching, or soreness in your vaginal area. Notify your doctor if you suspect a problem.

## Pre-labour contractions

Labour is an action of the uterus that begins slowly and then gathers speed and strength. After months of stretching larger, the uterus will finally start to contract in the weeks before birth. These Braxton Hicks contractions are usually painless, and should be irregular. Many mothers are unaware of them when they happen.

## Worries about labour

It is normal for you to have some worries about childbirth, especially if this is your first baby. In Canada, childbirth in a hospital setting is considered very safe. It is true that things can go wrong, but almost all babies are born normal and healthy. To return to the purpose of this handbook, research has shown that being prepared and learning about the birth process will make a real difference in labour. Women who have learned about labour and the birth process tend to be less frightened and anxious than women who have not. When there are fewer surprises, you will feel more confident and less anxious, and the pain will feel more manageable.

## Overdue babies

About 10 percent of women will not have delivered their babies by the end of their 41st week, or within one week after their due date. When a pregnancy lasts beyond 41 weeks it is called post-term and the babies are said to be overdue. To be sure your pregnancy is truly post-term, your baby's due date must be accurate. Your due date should have been calculated early in your pregnancy using the dates of your last menstrual period and the results of the ultrasound that may have been done around your 16th to 20th week. Trying to calculate due dates late in pregnancy using uncertain menstrual dates or late ultrasounds is not reliable.

### An aging placenta

A small percentage of overdue babies will develop health problems. We don't know why a few overdue babies have these problems, but it may be because of an aging placenta. The placenta deteriorates as it gets older, and it can begin to lose its ability to do its job. When this happens, it may mean that fewer nutrients and less blood and oxygen will reach your baby. In some cases, this can cause your baby's growth to slow down.

## Keeping your overdue baby safe

If your baby is still not born after your 41st week, or within a week after your due date, you and your doctor will face a decision—to monitor the baby closely while awaiting the start of labour, or to induce labour.

There are several ways to monitor your overdue baby's health while you wait. Induction of labour is described on page 93.

COUNTING THE BABY'S MOVEMENTS—One of the best ways to determine if your overdue baby is active is to count the number of movements he makes. You can do "movement counts" at home, at any time of the day. You are the best judge of whether your baby is moving the same as he was before. Remember that overdue babies feel very crowded and their movements may not be as vigorous. But no matter what, you should still feel movement throughout the day, every day. You may be asked to write down your baby's movement counts.

ULTRASOUND TESTING—An ultrasound may be done to help doctors determine the health of your baby. The results of this test are often compared to any previous ultrasounds you may have had.

NON-STRESS TEST—A non-stress test is a recording of your baby's heart rate, taken at your doctor's clinic or at the hospital. The rate is measured for 20 to 30 minutes, and if the baby is healthy, the recording will show accelerations in the fetal heart rate and movement.

At an appropriate point, your labour may be started for you (induced).

---

### 2. CHANGING OF THE CERVIX

TRUE
*Your cervix (the opening to your womb) begins to change—it begins to soften, shorten and open. The cervix opening to 3-4 cm is a sign of active labour.*

closed cervix                    open cervix

FALSE
*There is no change in your cervix. It doesn't soften, shorten, thin out or open up.*

---

### 3. REGULARITY OF CONTRACTIONS

TRUE
*The contractions usually become quite regular and predictable. Typically, contractions will last 30–70 seconds long, and will begin about five minutes apart (or less).*

FALSE
*The contractions are irregular, and never really settle down into a pattern.*

## RECORDING MY PROGRESS

Date:

Week of pregnancy:

Blood pressure:

Weight:

Fetal heart rate:

## THINGS TO DISCUSS WITH MY
## HEALTH CARE PROVIDER:

# My pregnancy journal
## 36 to 42 weeks

You will have prenatal examinations every week during the last 4-6 weeks. At each visit, you and your baby will be watched closely to make sure that you are both growing well, and that your body is continuing to prepare for the big event.

**Your time is here**

*After months of waiting (and possibly when you least expect it) you will start to feel the beginning of labour. The time to have your baby has finally arrived. Like most women, you may feel surprised, excited, and even a little scared.*

## When labour begins

It is believed that hormones play an important role in the start of labour, but no one knows for sure what really causes it. There is no way to predict exactly when your labour will begin.

### Signs of labour
Some women realize they are in labour right away, but others may not be so sure. Sometimes, it is even hard for the experts to tell. If you are in doubt, you should go to the hospital.

**Show**—A mucous plug has formed at the opening of your cervix during your pregnancy. When the cervix begins to open, this plug is released. You may notice a thick, unusual discharge from your vagina that may be blood-tinged, or notice an increase in vaginal discharge that is clear or pinkish. This may happen several days before labour starts—wait for further signs.

**Rupture of membranes**—When the sac full of amniotic fluid surrounding your baby springs a leak, or breaks completely, the membranes are said to be ruptured. This is often referred to as your "water breaking." It can happen several hours before labour, or at any time during labour. Go to the hospital if this happens.

**Contractions**—Labour often begins with contractions of the uterus, as your uterus tightens and then relaxes. These contractions open the cervix and push the baby down the birth canal. See pages 88-89 to help you tell the difference between true versus false labour.

Labour contractions are painful and regular, and usually last between 30 to 70 seconds long (see pages 88-89).

## When labour may be induced

An overdue baby is only one reason why labour may be induced. If your water breaks without labour starting on its own, you and your doctor will face the decision to induce labour or to wait for it to start on its own. Either course may be appropriate, depending on the situation. The decision may depend on factors such as how long the membranes have been ruptured, whether the cervix is ripe, the risk of infection, and your own feelings.

There are other reasons why it may be best to induce a pregnancy at term (40 weeks) or before, such as if the mother has high blood pressure that is worsening or an illness such as diabetes, if there are signs that the baby is not growing well, or if there are other medical concerns.

Labour should be induced only for these valid medical reasons.

### How labour is induced
There are several common ways to induce labour.

**Stripping the membranes**—The sac filled with amniotic fluid that surrounds your baby is attached to the inside of your cervix. It is a common and acceptable practice for your doctor to strip these membranes away from the cervix, without breaking through the membranes, in order to help ripen the cervix and prevent your pregnancy from being overdue. After discussions with you, your doctor will place a finger into your cervix (much like putting a finger into a small doughnut hole), and then circle the finger against the inside of the cervix to detach the membranes that are stuck to the sides. This routine and simple procedure is performed in your doctor's office, with your consent, usually some time after 38 weeks. After the procedure, most women experience a small amount of cramping that lasts a short time, along with a small amount of pinkish discharge.

**Ripening the cervix**—Normally, the cervix begins to soften, widen, and shorten before labour starts. This is called ripening. If your cervix is not getting ready for labour on its own, and you are having labour induced, your doctor may try to ripen your cervix. This is commonly done by placing a special gel or insert containing hormones (prostaglandin E2) onto your cervix, or into your vagina. Another method is to place a rubber tube with

*The number I should call when labour begins is:*

*Calling this number will put me in touch with:*

*I should go directly to the hospital if:*

*Any special instructions I should follow when I am in labour are:*

*Judge the situation and try to fit in. If she is quiet, you can be quiet.*

*Some labouring women don't like to be touched during contractions and others need to be.*

*She may need many words of encouragement, or very few.*

*If something you tried didn't work at one point during labour, try it again later. It may work then.*

*Always be positive and never criticize anything she does or wants.*

*When labour is very intense, some women say things they don't mean that may hurt your feelings. Try not to take it personally. It is the pain talking.*

*Keep the family updated by choosing one main person to call the others. Only this one person should call the hospital for information.*

*If the labour is long, make sure you get a bite to eat so you don't feel faint during the delivery.*

a balloon on the end into the cervix. The balloon is then inflated inside the cervix, which may cause ripening to take place. It is very important to soften or ripen the cervix before inducing labour.

**Rupturing the membranes**—If the membranes of the amniotic sac are still unbroken, the next step may be to break them, using a simple and almost painless procedure. For most women, labour will begin within 12 hours after rupturing the membranes, particularly if her cervix is ripe. Sometimes, the membranes may also be ruptured as a way to speed along a labour that was not induced, but began on its own.

**Starting the contractions**—Your body naturally produces a hormone called oxytocin, which is responsible for starting uterine contractions. Medical researchers have developed drugs that are identical to the hormone your body naturally produces. These synthetic drugs can be given intravenously to start contractions. When the dose is increased, the contractions become more frequent and stronger.

## Labour support

Most women find it very comforting to have a familiar face around them during labour. You can choose anyone you wish to be your labour coach—including the baby's father, a friend, a family member and/or a professional doula. Coaches can offer you the emotional support you need, rub your aching back if it helps, coach you to remember the special breathing techniques you learned in prenatal classes, and hold your hand when you need it most. Some hospitals have volunteers to help labouring mothers.

### A word about the labour coach's job

Studies show that women benefit in a number of ways if they have a supportive person who knows them to help them with their labour.

As a labour coach, especially if this is your first time, you may be wondering what you can do to help during labour. Some coaches worry they may feel queasy, or will be unable to offer enough support. But remember, there are many things you can do to help your partner during labour.

Before labour begins, encourage your partner to rest often, and take over her share of the cleaning, laundry, and cooking.

If you were involved in the preparation of the birthing plan, you know what type of birth experience she hopes for. She may ask you to be her voice to the staff during her labour.

It is helpful for you to remain as calm as possible and to keep your movements slow, quiet, and steady when you are with her. Be encouraging and offer her words of praise. Help her try to relax between contractions. When you assist with special breathing, allow her to follow her own rhythm (sometimes her body will tell her which rhythm is best; it may not be the pattern you learned and practised).

If she seems to lose control, remain close, talk her quietly through the contraction, keep eye contact, and try to get her back on track for the next one.

Be flexible about your birthing plan and don't feel upset if things don't go exactly the way you had planned. Listen carefully to your partner's wishes—they may change. Remember to take care of yourself during this long and stressful process. Take time to eat, drink, and rest.

**Your labour and delivery health care providers**
If you are planning to deliver your baby in a hospital, you will meet your obstetrical nurse when you arrive. Usually, labour and delivery professionals are registered nurses but some may have midwife qualifications. If possible, the same nurse will stay with you during your labour and delivery. Licensed midwives also care for women during pregnancy, labour, and delivery.

Studies show that you will benefit in a number of ways by having a nurse or midwife who is focused on your care. These partners are there to help you master techniques to make your labour easier. They are also very experienced, and know when the birth is progressing normally and how to recognize when something is not going well.

---

### GO TO THE HOSPITAL WHEN:

*Your water breaks in a gush or your water is leaking steadily.*

*Your contractions are regular and five minutes apart (and the hospital is less than 30 minutes away).*

*Your contractions are regular and 10 minutes apart (and the hospital is more than 30 minutes away).*

IF YOU ARE UNSURE, CALL THE  LABOUR AND DELIVERY UNIT AT YOUR HOSPITAL.

MONITORING YOUR BABY
DURING LABOUR

*If your pregnancy is considered a normal one, as most are, studies show the best way to check your baby during labour is by listening to the fetal heart through the mother's abdomen. Ideally, your nurse will check the fetal heart rate (FHR) often and regularly by using a stethoscope or a hand-held Doppler, a machine that picks up the sounds of your baby's heart.*

*The heart rate will be checked for a full minute after a contraction, about two to four times every hour during the first stage of labour. When you begin the second stage of labour, and start pushing, your nurse will check the heartbeat every five minutes.*

*Sometimes a machine is used to continuously read and record your baby's heartbeat and the length and strength of your contractions. This external monitor prints the information onto a continuous strip of paper that your health care professionals will be able to read. This monitor is attached to you by way of a simple belt worn around your belly.*

*(continued on sidebar page 97)*

## The stages of labour

There are four stages of labour. The first stage begins when the contractions start and become regular, and ends when your cervix is fully dilated (10 centimetres). The second stage of labour begins when your cervix is fully dilated and ends when your baby is born. The third stage of labour begins after the baby is born and ends when the placenta is delivered. The fourth stage of labour ends about two hours after the birth. The average labour lasts about 12–14 hours for first-time mothers, and second and subsequent labours are generally shorter. Keep in mind that these numbers are just averages, and that every labour is different.  No one can predict what your labour will be like, or how long it will last.

The first stage of labour is usually the longest stage of the labour process, and is divided into three parts: early, active, and transition.

Early in the pregnancy, your cervix is a thick-walled canal about 2.5 cm (one inch) long. During the last few weeks of your pregnancy, hormones will cause your cervix to soften. This is called the ripening of the cervix.

Once labour starts, contractions cause this ripened cervix to dilate, or open up, and to efface, or thin out. At the end of the first stage of labour, your cervix will be open 10 centimetres (four inches) and the sides will be very thin. At this point, your uterus, cervix, and vagina will be reshaped to form one long birth canal for the baby to pass through.

## The first stage of labour

### Early or latent stage of labour (0-3 cm)
In this early stage, it may be difficult to know for sure if you are in labour. Monitoring the strength and regularity of your contractions, and paying close attention for any changes to your cervix will help you and your health care provider know for sure (see pages 88-89).  If you go to the hospital during this stage, you will be assessed, and then either observed for a few hours in an assessment area or advised to go home until your labour really starts.

During this "latent" or "early" labour time, keep up your fluids and try a warm bath or shower. Sometimes, if you have been having irregular contractions and you are tired, you may be offered some pain medication to help you rest and regain your strength for when real labour begins.

### First stage—active—3-8 cm
In the active part of the first stage of labour, you will notice your contractions have become much stronger. They last about 45 seconds and occur about every 3–5 minutes. As the contractions progress, your cervix will continue to thin and open. At the end of this stage, your cervix should be eight centimetres open. You may begin to feel quite tired and anxious, making it very important to relax as much as you can between contractions. You may have back pain because of the position of the baby's head in your pelvis.

### First stage—transition—8-10 cm
You are coming down the home stretch now. Your contractions may be every 2–3 minutes and will usually last about 60–90 seconds. This helps your cervix to dilate fully, to 10 centimetres. In many women, however, the labour actually slows down during the transition stage, and it may take longer to dilate these final two centimetres. At the same time that this is occurring, the baby's head should be slowly going down into the pelvis.

*If your pregnancy or labour is considered high risk, or if a problem arises during labour, the health team may need to use some form of constant internal monitoring to get a good idea of how your baby is doing, particularly during the contractions. This type of monitoring may be necessary if your baby's heart rate is too slow or too fast, or if she has had a bowel movement, passing meconium (the first stool material) within the uterus.*

*Internal monitoring is done by attaching a scalp clip to a part of the baby that can be reached through the open cervix (usually the top of the head). This device reads and records the fetal heart rate (FHR). Sometimes it is necessary to take a sampling of blood from the baby's scalp so that her blood oxygen and pH levels can be checked (fetal scalp sampling).*

| | |

**WHEN THINGS ARE GOING SLOWLY**

*Slow progress in labour is common. The appropriate rate varies, depending on how many babies you have had. With a first baby, for example, the time from the beginning of active labour to delivery will average 12 hours. You may be given an infusion of oxytocin, a synthetic hormone, to make your contractions more effective, particularly when dilation is occurring very slowly and your contractions are not frequent or strong enough. In several large studies, this "active management" of labour has been shown to decrease the rate of caesarean delivery. It also prevents labour from going on for an abnormally long time.*

## Medication-free techniques to make labour easier

Labour tends to be easier if you are relaxed and confident, rather than tense and fearful. Many of the techniques that you and your support team use to make labour easier are geared toward helping you relax and remain in control of your body and your mind.

You and your labour coach will have learned and practised several different techniques in the weeks and months before labour began. Remember, a technique that works for other women may not necessarily work for you, so it's important to have as many techniques as possible at your disposal.

### Special breathing
Several special breathing techniques may help make your job easier and promote a sense of control over your body and mind. Sometimes you will follow your body's lead, and breathe in whatever manner feels right, but you may find some of the following techniques helpful.

### Slow breathing
This slow, deep breathing technique has been known to work best in the early stage of labour by shifting your attention away from the contractions. Begin by taking a deep breath through your nose or mouth. Then, purse your lips and very slowly blow the air out. Usually the rate and rhythm of this comes naturally, but the rate should be like counting in for 3-4 counts, out 3-4 counts. Many labouring women do this type of slow breathing throughout their entire labour and it works well for them.

### Light/quick breathing
This type of breathing has been known to work best during the active part of labour, when the contractions are coming more often and getting quite strong. When a contraction begins, start by breathing slowly in and out. As the contraction gets stronger, shorten your breaths. At the peak (strongest point) of the contraction, breathe lightly in and quickly out, making a puffing sound much like the panting of a dog. When the contraction starts to ease off, slow your breathing down again and then take a deep, cleansing breath.

**Transition breathing (pant-pant-blow)**
This type of breathing has been known to work best during the transition stage of labour when the labour is most intense and you may no longer be able to slow breathe. Transition breathing is commonly called pant-pant-blow breathing, and can help you avoid the urge to push against a cervix that is not fully dilated. It is done like this: take a deep breath in, then break your exhalation into two short pants, followed by a longer blow to empty your lungs.

## COPING WITH EARLY LABOUR

| You can: | Your labour coach can: |
|---|---|
| Tune into your body; go with the flow. | Have the car ready and filled with gas. |
| At night, try to sleep. | Put your bags into the car. |
| During the day, alternate activity with rest. | Help you relax, offer you back or foot massages. |
| Take a warm bath or shower (unless your water has broken or is leaking). | If necessary, let people know labour has started. |
| Walk with your labour coach or watch a movie. | Encourage you to walk, rest, eat, and drink. |
| Use relaxation techniques. | Time contractions from the beginning of one to the beginning of the next. |
| Breathe slowly and deeply through contractions. | Be calm and reassuring. |
| Keep your energy levels up by lightly eating and drinking. | Prepare you a light meal; offer you plenty of fluids. |

## COPING WITH ACTIVE LABOUR

### YOU CAN:

*Relax; go with the flow of contractions.*

*Use light/quick breathing or a slow relaxation breathing.*

*Change positions often; don't lie on your back; moving will speed labour.*

*Expect contractions to get much stronger after water breaks.*

*Ask for pain relief if you want it.*

*Use visualization to help you to focus.*

*Take a warm bath to relax.*

*Use a birthing ball to put counter-pressure on your perineum and to help open up your pelvis.*

*Ask for help; make your needs known.*

*Empty your bladder as needed.*

### YOUR LABOUR COACH CAN:

*Massage tense muscles.*

*Stay with you.*

*Help with your breathing, let your rhythm dictate the breathing pattern that is best for you.*

*Encourage and help you to change positions often. Use pillows for support. Walk with you. Help you to sit upright if you wish.*

*Apply firm counter-pressure to your back during contractions. Give back rubs between contractions.*

*Be your voice to the staff. Let you focus on labour.*

*Encourage you and tell you how far you have come. Help you get through contractions one at a time and prepare for the next one.*

*Support your choices. Never criticize. Make the room as peaceful as possible. Be calm and reassuring.*

## COPING WITH THE TRANSITION TO SECOND STAGE LABOUR

### YOU CAN:

*Move around as much as you need to get comfortable.*

*If your cervix is not 10 centimetres dilated, and you have the urge to push, try pant-pant-blow breathing to avoid pushing.*

*Get through contractions one at a time. Try to think of the pains as closer together, not stronger.*

*Take a shower or tub bath if possible.*

*Envision your body opening up like a flower to let your baby move out.*

*Wash hands and face with a cool cloth. Change your gown.*

*Suck ice chips or sip water to keep your mouth moist.*

*Tell your labour coach or nurse if you have the urge to push.*

### YOUR LABOUR COACH CAN:

*Support your choice of position.*

*Help with breathing. Maintain eye contact so that you feel connected to your labour coach and more in control.*

*Remind you labour's almost over; the baby's nearly out. Be calm, reassuring, and positive.*

*Rub tense muscles if you want, especially around the lower back where the baby's head may be applying pressure.*

*Help you with visualizations and relaxation.*

*Stroke your face, hair, or other part of your body if you like.*

*Offer ice chips; apply a cool cloth to your brow.*

*If you have the urge to push, help you to transition breathe (pant-pant-blow) to avoid pushing until the nurse comes.*

## Body positions

The position of your body can sometimes make labour easier. Many studies have been done to find out which positions are best for both you and your baby. You should feel free to labour in any position that makes your labour easier, and to change positions as often as you want. The use of pillows can be helpful to prop up your legs, arms, and belly. It is not a good idea to lie flat on your back during labour because the weight of the uterus may squeeze a large blood vessel against your spine, slowing the blood supply to the baby.

### Sitting upright

Sitting up straight (or leaning back very slightly) is the most common position for giving birth, and offers benefits for both you and your baby. Studies show this position may help your uterus to contract and, therefore, may shorten the second stage of your labour. In addition, this sitting position seems to help the baby move down the birth canal. Further studies show that babies born to mothers who were sitting upright during the actual delivery had better oxygen levels in their blood. Mothers reported they liked this position because it was easier to see their baby and easier to bond with the baby once it was born. Most hospitals have birthing beds that make this sitting position easier.

### Lying on your side

You may lie on your side at one time or another during labour but you may not have thought of actually delivering your baby while lying on your side. This position for birth is sometimes required because some women feel more comfortable labouring on their side. From a medical point of view, this position may help your doctor deliver your baby safely if you have certain heart conditions, hip joint problems, or varicose veins in your legs. Your labour coach will need to support your upper leg during the birth.

### Squatting—delivery only

The squatting position has two benefits. First, the squatting position makes bearing down (pushing) easier because the uterus is able to fall forward with the force of gravity. This helps your baby to move down the birth canal. Second, studies show squatting helps to widen your pelvis, allowing more room for the baby to move down and out. North American women sometimes find this position uncomfortable because they are not used to it. Some hospitals provide birthing bars on their birthing beds to help women who choose to use this position.

### Kneeling on all fours—usually for delivery, or sometimes late in the first stage

This position is a reasonable option for some women. Very few studies have been done of this position. Some experts believe it may help a baby turn around into the proper position for delivery if it hasn't done so on its own. Many women rock back and forth on all fours during contractions to help relieve their backache. This may be a useful position to try.

### Hydrotherapy

Aside from giving comfort, there is good evidence that hydrotherapy (using showers, whirlpool baths, and tub baths) is beneficial to labouring women. Although hydrotherapy doesn't seem to shorten labour, it does seem to reduce a woman's stress. When a woman has less stress, more endorphins seem to be present in her body. Endorphins are the body's "feel good" hormone. In addition, less stress allows levels of the hormone oxytocin to rise in the body. This extra oxytocin helps the contractions to become more regular and stronger.

Before you begin water therapy, it is best to get help from your nurse. The water should not be too hot, as this can dilate the blood vessels found close to your skin, causing your blood pressure to drop. This may make you feel dizzy.

If you spend a long time in the tub, it is important to drink fluids or to suck on ice chips so that you don't become dehydrated. It is still important to empty your bladder as needed, but be very careful getting in and out of a slippery tub. During water therapy, your baby's heart rate will still need to be counted every now and then by your nurse. While in the tub, labouring mothers and their labour coaches can also try some of the other techniques that make labour easier, such as touch and massage therapy, visualization, and special breathing.

Hydrotherapy is usually limited to the first stage of labour.

### Transcutaneous Electric Nerve Stimulation (TENS)

TENS is a safe, medication-free, non-invasive way to manage pain. It can help relieve pain by sending small electrical impulses through electrodes placed on the skin (on the belly or back) to the nerve fibres under the skin. TENS is believed to work in two different ways. First, the electrical impulses block a pain signal from being carried to the brain. The contractions may be causing pain, but your brain doesn't sense it. Secondly, TENS is also thought to work by triggering your body to release more endorphins—the body's "feel good" hormone.

If this method interests you, the physical therapy department of a hospital generally arranges TENS treatments. It may be beneficial to contact them before your labour, or to speak with your doctor about this method during a prenatal visit.

### Vocalization

You may worry that you will cry out loudly during labour. Some women do and others don't. Nurses and doctors are very used to hearing and seeing labouring women use these methods to cope with the stress of labour. Many women vocalize during labour, others chant, moan, rock their bodies or heads from side to side, or cry. These are perfectly normal ways to cope with labour and you should never feel embarrassed if you feel the need to use these methods.

## Using medication for pain relief

Two main types of medications are used to control pain during labour: painkillers or freezing. Painkillers are also known as analgesics. These medications dull the overall pain but do not cause a loss of feeling. Medications that "freeze" your body are called anesthetics. These medications cause a total loss of feeling in a certain area of the body. It is a good idea to talk about the kind of pain relief you would like in your birthing plan.

### Painkillers (analgesics)

Most powerful painkillers are narcotics. Examples of narcotics you may be offered are meperidine (Demerol®) or morphine. Narcotics are usually given by an injection into the muscles of the hip, or sometimes through an intravenous (IV) line. They dull the pain and make you feel sleepy, so that you can rest between contractions.  However, they can cross through the placenta and may make your baby sleepy as well.

To ensure there is time for the effects of narcotics to wear off before the baby is born, narcotics are usually given in the early and active stages of your labour. In this way, your baby will be born alert and active. But if your baby is born sleepy because of a pain shot you needed, the doctors and nurses can safely give the baby an antidote called Narcan® that will quickly waken the baby.

### Epidurals

An epidural block is a common procedure for giving an anesthetic medication to block the pain of labour and birth. In this procedure, a needle is inserted into a small space between the bones of your spine, and medication is injected into the space around the bundles of nerve endings found there. The medication numbs the nerves in that area and therefore blocks pain messages from going to your brain.

When the doctor puts the medication in place the first time, he will leave behind a small plastic tube (catheter) in the space between the bones, which will then be taped securely to the outside of your body. By doing this, your doctor is able to give you more of the medication if it is needed, without having to poke through your skin again with a needle.

Usually, the doctor will use this catheter to hook you up to a pump that will deliver the medication a bit at a time. If you wish to use this type of pain control, it is best to discuss this with your doctor before you go into labour.

The medication in epidurals can be delivered so that you can continue to have some control over your legs, labour in some different positions and be able to be up to go to the bathroom. This is called a "light" or "walking" epidural.  This is preferable because you can benefit from the positive effects of upright posture on the progress of labour.  You may also be able to feel the urge to push and push more effectively if you are not "frozen" from your epidural. Talk to your doctor (anesthetist) about this option.

## The second stage of labour

The cervix is now open 10 centimetres, or fully dilated. The baby is now ready to be pushed down the birth canal. During the second stage of labour, the contractions usually slow to 2–5 minutes apart and last about 45–90 seconds. This gives your body a well-needed rest period between contractions.

### Pushing

Most women feel an urge to push when their baby reaches a certain point in their pelvis. Pushing offers some relief from the "pressure" of labour. Pushing through a contraction has been described as a powerful release of stored energy that comes from deep within a woman's body and mind. You may feel empowered, strengthened, and in control when you begin to push.

Some women, particularly if they have had an epidural, don't feel the urge to push and may need extra help and coaching to push their baby out.

### When not to push
You may be asked to try not to push if your cervix is not quite ready (only 8–9 centimetres), or if your baby has not quite settled into the best position for pushing. However, sometimes the urge to push is so overpowering you are not able to resist it. With your nurse at your side to help you, you may be asked to put your knees very close to your chest and to use the pant-pant-blow method of special breathing until your cervix is completely open.

### No urge to push
Some women go through a short period in which they don't have any contractions or their contractions are very light and they have no urge to push. This has been called the "rest and be thankful" period.

If your cervix is fully dilated but you don't feel an urge to push yet, relax and rest for a bit. The urge will come in time. Sometimes, epidurals can affect a woman's ability to push, or can inhibit the urge to push. Your nurse or doctor will give you support and advice.

### The natural rhythm of pushing
There is no right or wrong way to push. Although it is still common to be encouraged to "take a deep breath in, hold it, and give one long steady hard push," studies show that this may not be the best method after all.

When women push naturally (i.e., without any instructions) they tend to do three to five short pushes during each contraction. As the second stage of labour moves along, the number of pushes per contraction tends to increase. With natural pushing, women take in several big breaths of air with each pushing effort, and slowly blow all the air out of their lungs. Studies show that the natural way of pushing ensures the most oxygen reaches your baby during the second stage of labour. Sometimes this natural way of pushing may take a few minutes longer. This can benefit you by allowing your skin more time to stretch, reducing the risk of tearing or needing an episiotomy. A slow, controlled journey down the birth canal is easier on the baby.

## Management of the delivery

In many cases, the delivery occurs without tearing. The birth attendant may attempt to massage the skin around the perineum, encouraging it to stretch. About 70 percent of first-time mothers will need some kind of small and simple repair to their perineum after childbirth. When the tears are repaired, the doctor may need to freeze the area with a local anesthetic to make it more comfortable. Research has shown that such small tears heal better, with less pain, than an episiotomy incision.

In some cases, it may be necessary to do an episiotomy if more room is needed to deliver the baby's head and shoulders, or if it is important to speed up the delivery because of concern for the baby.

An episiotomy is an incision about 2.5–5 centimetres (1–2 inches) long, made to the bottom of your vagina (perineum) toward the rectum or off to one side. Before making the incision, the doctor will freeze the area with a local anesthetic.

Episiotomies should be done only if necessary, depending on the situation at the time of the birth.

## Special delivery: complications in labour and delivery

### Breech babies
Most babies lie with their heads down in the birth canal. The first part of the baby that can be felt in the birth canal is called the "presenting part." The presenting part in a normal delivery is the head. When a baby is breech, the head is up and the buttocks are down. In this case, the presenting part is the buttocks. This is called a frank breech. Sometimes one foot or both feet hang lower than the buttock and the foot (or feet) would be the presenting part. This is called a footling or incomplete breech.

If you are near your due date (last 4-6 weeks) and a breech baby is suspected, an ultrasound will be done to confirm the position, size, and health of your baby.  If the baby is confirmed to be breech, two choices will be discussed with you.  The first option is to have a caesarean section instead of a vaginal delivery. The second option is a procedure known as external cephalic version. The doctor presses on your abdomen, turning the baby in a somersault so that you can try to have a vaginal delivery. Your health care provider will discuss these options with you. They are based on scientific studies, which show this is the safest way to handle a breech baby.

### Assisted births: forceps or vacuum extraction

Sometimes a baby needs to be helped from the birth canal. A doctor may choose to assist the birth using forceps or a vacuum extraction.

The most common reason for an assisted birth is a prolonged second stage of labour, when the mother is fatigued and can no longer push, and the baby is low enough to be delivered vaginally with a little help. Another reason for an assisted birth is that, if a baby's heartbeat has slowed, the baby may be in trouble.

Both forceps and vacuum extractor methods are common, safe, and very useful. Forceps are two slim, curved blades designed to slide around the baby's head inside the birth canal. Once they are in place, the doctor is able to gently pull the baby down and out with each contraction. There are several styles of forceps.

A better description of a vacuum-extraction-assisted birth might be a suction-assisted birth. In this case, a plastic cup, which is held in place by suction, is placed on top of the baby's head. A handle is attached to the cup, which enables the doctor to gently pull the baby down and out.

### Caesarean births

A caesarean section (also called a caesarean birth or a c-section) is the medical term for the surgical delivery of your baby from your uterus. In Canada, about 22 percent of women have caesarean births. Sometimes, for medical reasons, this surgery is scheduled and done before labour actually begins. At other times, if complications arise for the mother or the baby during labour, it is done when labour is already in progress.

FORCEPS ASSISTANCE

SUCTION ASSISTANCE

The most common reason for a caesarean is "failure to progress in labour." Despite good and regular contractions, the cervix stops dilating for several hours or the baby fails to descend into the pelvis for delivery. In these cases, and when other medical interventions have been tried without success (see page 109), a caesarean is necessary.

Concern about the baby's well-being is the second most common reason for a c-section. Usually, the concern is raised by changes in the baby's heart rate during labour, and is ideally confirmed with a fetal scalp blood sample. If either or both raise a strong suspicion that the baby may not be tolerating labour, and if the birth is not imminent, a c-section will be considered.

The third most common reason for a caesarean is the mother's previous childbirths by c-section. It used to be said that "once a caesarean, always a caesarean." However, this is no longer true. In fact, about 60–80 percent of women who previously had a caesarean birth will be able to deliver vaginally.

If you have had a c-section before, it is important for you to know that you have an excellent chance of having a normal delivery. Studies have shown that many women do not want to try labour again because they are afraid of another long painful labour that will only end in another c-section. If this is how you feel, discuss this with your doctor. You need to be reassured that you will have adequate pain relief.

Other less common reasons for c-sections include breech presentation (page 108), or bleeding from a separated placenta or from a placenta located over the cervix. Sometimes a c-section is needed to preserve the health of the mother, as in the case of serious illness such as toxemia or severe cases of diabetes. If a mother has an active herpes infection or is HIV positive, the baby will be delivered by c-section to prevent the disease from being transmitted to the baby during the birth.

Childbirth is an unpredictable experience that no one can fully control, no matter how prepared they may be. Whether you deliver your baby vaginally or by c-section, the goal of pregnancy is for you to become the mother of a healthy child. How you get to that goal is not as important as the goal itself. Childbirth is unpredictable, so you should be aware that a c-section is a possibility. For this reason, it may be a good idea to include a section in your birth plan that deals with what you would like to do if you need to have a caesarean birth.

Many healthy babies are delivered by caesarean birth to parents thankful this safe alternative for birthing exists. The possible need for an emergency caesarean birth is also another good reason to deliver your baby in the safety of a hospital setting.

## The third stage of labour

This stage of labour begins after the baby has been born and ends when the placenta emerges. Other than having a few mild contractions to help push out your placenta, your work is done, and this is a time of relief.

As long as your uterus continues to shrink and stays firm (and if there is no unusual bleeding), it is best to take a watch-and-wait approach to the delivery of the placenta. Usually, the placenta will emerge within 30 minutes after the birth.

If you need any repairs to your skin from tearing or an episiotomy, they will be done once the placenta has been delivered. Finally, to help encourage your uterus to shrink, and therefore help to stop the bleeding, your health care provider is likely to give you an injection of oxytocin, a synthetic hormone. Studies have shown that routine use of this hormone with the birth of the baby significantly reduces the amount of blood that a woman can lose after birth and can prevent postpartum hemorrhage (excessive bleeding).

During this time, your nurse will feel the size and shape of your uterus often to make sure it continues to shrink and the bleeding continues to slow down. Nurses will also be caring for your baby during this stage. You may tremble, feel chilled, or even a bit nauseated. The nausea should quickly pass and a warmed blanket will soothe your chills.

---

### THE THIRD STAGE OF LABOUR

YOU CAN:

Relax. Hold and touch your baby.

Provide skin-to-skin contact.

If you are shaky or chilled, ask for a warmed blanket.

Help push out the placenta when asked (it is not painful).

---

YOUR LABOUR COACH CAN:

Bond with the baby.

Help you get set up to breastfeed.

Offer you something to drink, wipe your face and hands with a damp cloth.

## APGAR SCORES

*A simple and quick method of testing newborns to see how fit and healthy they are is done one minute after the birth and again five minutes later. This test, called an Apgar Score, was developed by a paediatrician named Dr. Virginia Apgar. It is a very important and useful tool to help doctors determine if your baby will need special care after the birth. Five areas are rated during an Apgar Score test: the baby's heart rate, breathing, muscle tone, reflexes, and skin colour. Depending on how the baby is responding, each area is rated and given a number ranging from zero to two (with zero being the poorest response and two being the best response). The total number is the Apgar Score. Most babies score between 7 and 10.*

▶ *A baby who was born with a heart rate of 140 (scores 2), and a good strong cry (scores 2), with some movements (scores 1), coughing (scores 2) and pink all over (scores 2) will have an Apgar score of 9. Any score over 7 at 5 minutes predicts a healthy baby.*

### Cord blood gases

Immediately after birth, a "cord blood gases" test is done. This test is done by taking a sample of blood from a section of the umbilical cord after it has been cut. The blood's oxygen level and the blood's pH level are checked. The pH level is used to measure the balance of chemicals in the blood, and is an important measure of the baby's well-being at birth.

## The fourth stage of labour

The fourth stage of labour begins after the placenta is out and lasts about two hours. It is a time to rest, enjoy, and recover. During this time, you will be watched very closely for any problems that may arise. Your nurse will check your blood pressure, heart rate, breathing, the position of the top of your uterus, and the amount of bleeding from your vagina. It is during this stage, as both you and your baby adjust to the changes of childbirth, that you will have an important chance to bond with your baby.

| Apgar scores | | | |
|---|---|---|---|
| | score 0 | score 1 | score 2 |
| Heart rate | Absent | Slow (< 100 per minute) | 100 per minute |
| Breathing | Absent | Weak | Good, strong cry |
| Muscle tone | Limp | Some movements | Active movements |
| Reflexes | No response | Grimace, whimpering | Cough or sneeze |
| Skin colour | Blue or pale | Body pink, arms and legs blue | Completely pink |

## Bonding with your baby

You probably began to care deeply for your baby before she was born. Fathers can bond just as deeply as mothers, and should be given the chance to bond with their newborn within minutes after the birth. Some people feel love for their babies right away. For others, loving their baby takes time.

Studies show it is best for you and your baby not to be separated after the birth, unless there is a medical reason to do so. Consider keeping your baby unwrapped on your bare chest and abdomen, so that you have skin-to-skin contact during this time. This allows time for you to bond, to get to know each other. Bonding plays a very important role in helping you form a lifelong attachment to your baby.

Obstetrical nurses understand the bonding process and will encourage you. They will dim the lights, so the baby can open her eyes. Hold your baby closely, a few inches from your face so the newborn can see you. Talk quietly and softly using your normal tone of voice. You may notice the baby's face turning toward the sound of your voice and her eyes searching to make contact with yours. Over the next few days, take advantage of every chance you get to talk to your baby. Hold her close and continue to get as much skin-to-skin contact as you can. Handle a newborn slowly and feed her whenever she seems hungry.

For the first hour or two after the birth, both mother and baby are very alert, so this is an optimum time for both bonding and the first breastfeeding. Allow your baby to rest peacefully and give her time to adapt to the new surroundings. Within a few days, you two will know each other better. Within a few weeks, your new baby will know the world is a good and safe place to be.

## Postpartum hemorrhage

Bleeding too much after the birth (postpartum hemorrhage) happens to about 7–10 out of every 100 women. It can be quite worrisome. For the most part, uncontrolled bleeding happens for two reasons: a uterus that will not contract, or retained placenta fragments.

In the past, women died of this complication, but with modern medical care, postpartum hemorrhage is usually easy to stop. Postpartum hemorrhage is more common if: the baby was large, the labour long and difficult, there were multiple births (twins or more).

When the placenta separates from the inside wall of the uterus, blood vessels are left open-ended and leaking. The body's way of closing these blood vessels is to make the uterus clamp down tightly, squeezing them closed. The most common reason for uncontrolled bleeding after birth is a soft uterus that doesn't clamp down fast enough or hard enough to seal off these open blood vessels. If this is the cause of the bleeding, medication must be used to stimulate the uterus to contract in order to stop the bleeding.

The placenta should come out in one piece. If it breaks apart and pieces of the placenta stay inside the uterus, the pieces are "retained." This is the second most likely cause for bleeding after birth. When this happens, even the normal clamping and sealing off of the blood vessels by the uterus is not enough to stop the bleeding. If the placenta cannot be completely removed, you may need an operation (a D&C) right away to remove the retained pieces of placenta from the inside of the uterus.

### Preventing postpartum hemorrhage

It is best to try to prevent postpartum hemorrhage before it starts. Recent studies show that giving women hormone-like medications (oxytocin) can prevent the risk of postpartum hemorrhage by up to 40 percent. Because of this benefit, most hospitals now give these medications routinely, either during the second or third stage of labour. The medications are given by injection into a muscle, or into your vein.

Breastfeeding and massaging a soft uterus are two other valuable ways to prevent postpartum bleeding because both stimulate the uterus to contract.

## How long will you stay in hospital?

### Benefits of going home early

The length of time a new mother and her baby stay in the hospital after the birth has become much shorter over recent years. Although some of this change has been related to reduction in spending on health care, going home early can be better for both of you. Providing your baby is healthy and that you will have plenty of support at home, and if your hospital offers a follow-up home care program, you will probably be discharged 24–48 hours after the birth. Studies show that by going home soon after the birth of your healthy baby, you are more likely to adjust better to being a new mom. Your home is quieter and more relaxed than the hospital and you will probably sleep better in your own bed. Efforts to breastfeed may be more successful in the familiar comfort of your own home, and your baby is less likely to get an infection. Most importantly, it is easier for the baby's father and the rest of the family to spend time with the newest member of the family at home.

The maternity nurses are experts in teaching new mothers ways to care for their newborn babies. It is always a good idea to learn what you can from them during your hospital stay. Don't be shy about asking all the questions you have about anything, even if you think the question may be unimportant.

### Follow-up home care

In Canada, we are fortunate to have a public health system that provides follow-up home care after birth. This can vary from province to province. If you are going home early, it is very important that there be early follow-up of the baby, preferably with a home visit from a nurse or midwife.

---

### FOLLOW-UP HOME CARE INFORMATION

*Public health clinic phone number:*

_____

*First visit date and time:*

_____

_____

*Second visit date and time:*

_____

_____

*Public health nurse's name:*

_____

*Things I need to ask the public health nurse during my home visit:*

1. _____

2. _____

3. _____

4. _____

5. _____

The Society of Obstetricians and Gynaecologists of Canada and the Canadian Paediatric Society have issued a combined statement of the ways to know when it is safe for mothers and babies to leave the hospital early. They recommend early home follow-up as essential to early discharge. Visit www.sogc.org

The most important reason for this is to make sure feeding is well established, the baby is getting adequate fluid and nutrition in her first days, and to check for jaundice.

During a home visit, the nurse or midwife will examine you and your baby and will answer all your questions about caring for yourself and your newborn. This visit usually includes discussions about your body, breastfeeding, diapering, bathing, bonding with your baby, having sex again, birth control, and any other topic you feel a need to ask questions about. This private and close care is proving to be a very good way to give new mothers the confidence they need to look after their new babies. It is a good idea to write your questions down before the nurse arrives so that you will remember what you wanted to ask.

**Longer hospital stays**
Sometimes, it is best to stay in the hospital a little longer than usual. This may be the case if there were problems during the birth, if you had a long labour, or if you or your baby needs special care or rest. In addition, a longer hospital stay may be important if your hospital does not offer a community-based home care program or if you do not have enough support at home. Talk to your obstetrical nurse or your doctor if you have concerns about going home.

## If things don't go well for your baby

Most babies are born perfect in every way. Despite advances in modern medicine, babies are sometimes born seriously ill or with birth defects. Very rarely, babies die. All parents hope for the best during pregnancy and most have bonded deeply with their unborn child before the birth. They begin to think of their baby as a person, as the newest member of their family.

It is a great shock when a baby is born with birth defects or without signs of life. Many mothers feel their bodies have betrayed them, that their bodies have let everyone down, including the baby and their partner. Some worry they did something to cause the birth defect or loss of life. This is almost never true.

Parents can feel a deep sense of loss even if the baby is born alive but with serious birth defects or an illness. They grieve for the child with whom they cannot share a normal life.

The deepest and most profound sense of loss comes with the death of a baby. Many parents, understandably, have trouble coping with their loss. Such a sudden tragedy causes intense sadness, shock, disbelief, and anger.

For parents and family, the grieving process is a necessary part of healing. Grieving helps parents cope. All parents need bereavement support at such a tragic time in their lives.

## Say goodbye to your baby

You can help create memories of your baby by giving yourself a chance to hold him and say goodbye. If your baby died because of birth defects, you may be afraid to see him, but in almost all cases, what the parents imagine is worse than it really is.

You may want to have a memorial service or funeral, or you may choose a private ceremony. As grieving parents, you need to be able to talk about your feelings. Your baby is a real part of your life.

Nurses have done studies that show that parents need bereavement support to help them deal with their grief, so many hospitals have a process available to grieving parents.

### YOU AND YOUR PARTNER

*Your relationship with your partner may suffer from the loss. You may find you have trouble talking to one another and cannot face each other. You may find it hard to do the normal things you used to do. It may be hard to start making love again. You may have unresolved feelings of anger at the other person and you may not know why. You may be searching for someone to blame. It is normal to feel this way.*

*Be patient with each other. Tell each other how you are feeling and be as open and honest as you can. Seek professional counselling. If your partner can't talk about the baby's death right now, remind yourself that you will be able to talk to each other about it in the future. Your baby is not forgotten. Everyone grieves in their own way and at their own pace.*

*Make an extra effort to be tender toward your partner. Be reassuring to each other, use touch to show you care. Your baby was conceived out of your love for each other. Hold tight to the memories of your lives together before tragedy struck and know that some day peace will find you again.*

BABY'S BIRTHDAY

## My baby's journal

Date:

Time of birth:

Weight:

Length:

Hair colour:

Eye colour:

Health care providers:

Notes:

CHAPTER SEVEN

Taking care of yourself

## RECIPE FOR REST

Many new mothers have a burst of energy right after their babies are born, and then feel very tired. Your baby will be hungry every 2–3 hours or so for the first little while, and it may seem as though the feeding cycle never really ends. This is perfectly normal, but it does take a great deal of energy to keep up such a busy schedule. It is very important to get enough rest. Sleep when the baby sleeps. We'll say that again... It is very important to get enough rest.

### HERE IS AN EASY RECIPE TO REMEMBER:

**R** Relax whenever you can. Take a nap, read, watch television and, again, sleep when the baby sleeps!

**E** Eat well and drink plenty of fluids, especially if you are breastfeeding.

**S** Share the responsibility of your new baby with your partner, family, and friends. Ask for help.

**T** Take the time to enjoy the baby. Cuddle, coo, sing to your baby. Let the housework wait.

---

*One of the most important things you can do for your new baby is to take care of yourself. It is easier to look after a newborn if you are rested and healthy. You will need time to get used to all the changes having a baby brings. Your body has gone through many changes during pregnancy, and now you are not pregnant any more. That alone is a lot to get used to. Getting back to the way you were before pregnancy takes time. This is a good time to ask for the help of family and friends or to accept their offers to help cook meals, clean house, do laundry, or babysit other children.*

## Your changing body (postpartum)

The many changes your body went through during pregnancy took place over more than nine months. Realistically, it will take about the same amount of time for things to return to normal, so be patient with yourself. After delivery, your uterus is round and hard. It is about 17.5 centimetres long (seven inches) and can be felt in the lower abdomen. Six weeks after the birth, your uterus will be about 7.5 centimetres (three inches) long and you won't be able to feel it any more by pressing on your abdomen. Breastfeeding helps the uterus to shrink back to its normal size more quickly.

The area between your rectum and your vagina is called your perineum. It will have stretched during the delivery. Your perineum may feel swollen, bruised, and tender. You may have stitches from a tear or episiotomy. These stitches will dissolve over time, but they can be itchy while they heal. Continue with your Kegel exercises (page 46) after six weeks. They will help the stretched muscles in your perineum regain their tone. Some women experience a sensation of numbness in their perineum, which passes over time.

## The baby blues

After giving birth, it is normal to cry for no reason, to feel anxious, frightened, and sad. More than 70 percent of all new mothers feel a little depressed after the baby is born. This mild depression is thought to be linked to the changing levels of pregnancy hormones. It may also be linked to feelings of loss, since the baby is no longer inside you. Usually the baby blues start within a couple of days of the birth. They may last for hours or days. Normally, they go away within two weeks without any treatment.

You may feel a wide range of changing emotions. One minute you feel happy, the next minute you feel sad. You may feel very tired, then get a burst of energy. You may have trouble sleeping or making decisions. You may feel confident, then insecure. You may feel as though you will never get your life back or your body back into shape. You may feel tired all the time and may not be interested in sex at all. All of these feelings are completely normal. Now is the perfect time to reach out to your partner, family, and friends for love, support, and help.

### When "the blues" turn into depression

If the baby blues seem to be getting worse instead of better, or if they last more than two weeks, you may be developing postpartum depression. This happens to a small number of new mothers. Your feelings of sadness have turned to deep despair and a sense of hopelessness. You may resent being on call 24 hours a day, every day. You may love all the attention the baby gets and feel jealous at the same time. You may feel in charge and then angry that you are in charge. You may begin to question your ability to look after your baby. You may feel very frustrated and even angry when your baby cries, that the baby is crying just to annoy you. You may think about harming the baby or yourself, and may even tell yourself the feelings you are having are not normal. If you are feeling this way, get help right away. Treatment is available for postpartum depression. Talk to your public health nurse, your doctor or your midwife about your feelings.

## Normal vaginal discharge

The vaginal discharge after birth is called lochia. It is made up of blood and tissue from the lining of the uterus. The lochia is bright red at first and may contain a few small clots. Bright red blood may flow again for short periods during or after breastfeeding. This is normal, and due to mild contractions of the uterus caused by breastfeeding. If blood has had a chance to collect

### RECOGNIZING SIGNS OF POSTPARTUM DEPRESSION

*If any of these apply to you, get help.*

- *My baby blues haven't gone away after two weeks.*
- *I have strong feelings of sadness or guilt.*
- *I often feel very anxious.*
- *I have strong feelings of hopelessness or helplessness.*
- *I can't sleep, even when tired.*
- *I sleep all the time, even when my baby is awake.*
- *I am not able to eat, even when hungry.*
- *I am not able to eat because I am never hungry or because I feel sick.*
- *I worry about the baby too much; I'm obsessed about him.*
- *I don't worry about the baby at all; it's almost like I don't care.*
- *I am having panic attacks.*
- *I have feelings of anger toward the baby.*
- *I think about harming my baby or myself.*

*If you have any of these signs, get help right away. If you know a new mother who has these signs of depression, get help for her. Counselling and treatment will help the feelings go away. Don't wait; call your doctor, midwife or public health nurse.*

## SIGNS OF BLEEDING PROBLEMS

*It is not normal for your flow to stay heavy or become heavier. Normally, you would notice that your flow is gradually decreasing with each passing day. If your flow has been slowing down, and suddenly you develop a lot of heavy, bright red blood (which soaks through one or more maxi-pads within two hours and does not slow or stop with rest), do not wait, go to the hospital immediately.*

*In addition, it is not normal for you to develop large blood clots. It is also abnormal to notice an unusual discharge or foul smell coming from your vagina. If this happens, it may mean you have developed a vaginal infection or an infection at the site of your episiotomy. This can be serious and you should call your doctor right away. You may need antibiotics. If your flow has not completely stopped after six weeks, make an appointment to see your doctor.*

in the vagina while you are lying down, it can gush out for a short time when you stand up. This is also normal for the first few days. Within a few days, your flow will begin to decrease and will become darker. As your flow decreases, it is normal to notice occasional blood spotting. Eventually, your flow will turn whitish or yellow and gradually stop. The overall length of time a woman flows can vary from 10 days to five weeks. If you are a second-time mother, your flow may not be the same as it was with your last baby.

If your flow is heavier than you think is normal, is heavier than a period, or the smell is foul, check with your doctor. It is best to use sanitary pads, not tampons.

## Having sex again

When to have sex again is a personal choice. It is safe to do so once the bleeding has stopped but you should have sex again only when you feel ready. You should not let yourself feel rushed into having sex. Your body, mind, and spirit need time to adjust to the changes childbirth and motherhood bring. If you are like most new mothers, you will probably use all the energy you have to look after the baby. You may feel quite tired for the first few weeks.

You may worry that sexual intercourse may be painful. If it is, special jellies or creams are helpful to lubricate the vagina. You can also try changing positions to see if one is more comfortable than another. You may feel mildly depressed and uninterested in sex. Some new mothers feel insecure about their changed body image and may not feel attractive for the first little while. All of these feelings and worries are completely normal.

Some men don't feel like having sex too soon after the baby is born, either. They too may feel a bit worn out by late-night feedings, all the excitement, and their added sense of responsibility. Most men recognize that you need the time to recover from the birth, both emotionally and physically.

Most couples don't have sex for weeks; some don't have sex for months. This does not mean your relationship is in trouble. It only means that you are both taking time to adjust to the changes a baby brings. It is very important to trust each other and talk about your feelings. There are many non-sexual ways to show your partner how you feel. If you have any concerns about resuming sexual relations with your partner, make an appointment with your doctor for a checkup. For a discussion of birth control choices, see pages 126-128.

## Common discomforts after giving birth

### Tender breasts

When your milk comes in, about 2-4 days after the baby is born, your breasts may become very full, sore, and hard (see page 142 for a discussion of engorgement). If you are breastfeeding, feed your baby often to help drain the milk glands. Warmed towels applied to your breasts may be soothing.

If you are not breastfeeding, ice packs may help reduce the swelling, but do not empty or pump your breast as this will only cause more milk to be produced. If you are not breastfeeding, take pain medication. Good support is important when your breasts are tender, and it helps to wear a well-fitting support bra, even at night.

### Vaginal pain

It is normal for the perineum (the area around your anus and vagina) to be swollen, bruised, and tender after you have given birth. For some women, this soreness lasts up to six weeks. If you have stitches, you may feel even more discomfort. Try this: dampen and freeze a clean maxi-pad. Put the frozen pad in your underwear. This should help reduce swelling. Sometimes a warm bath helps relieve the itching caused by healing stitches. Keep the vaginal area clean to avoid infection. Get plenty of rest with your feet up to take the pressure off your bottom. If you need it, take pain medication.

### Cramping

Pains that feel like strong menstrual cramps are called afterpains. They are caused by the uterus as it shrinks. Afterpains may be worse during breastfeeding. First-time mothers may not feel afterpains. Try taking a warm bath, or put a heating pad across your abdomen. Pain medication sometimes helps, particularly those medications meant for menstrual cramps. The deep breathing and relaxation techniques you learned during pregnancy may also help.

### Bowel movements

It is perfectly normal if you do not have a bowel movement for 2–3 days after the birth of your baby. Your bowel is sluggish if you haven't eaten much or if you've received painkillers. In addition, the abdominal muscles that help push out a bowel movement are stretched and not as effective.

Many women fear the first bowel movement will be painful because of hemorrhoids or a bruised perineum. For this reason, they may "hold back" having a bowel movement. Try not to do this. Holding back may make your stool hard. Instead, do what you can to avoid hard stools. Drink plenty of fluids and fruit juice, and eat foods high in fibre, such as bran muffins, bran cereal, fresh fruit, and vegetables. Stool softeners with psyllium or natural fibre are available at the drugstore. Hard, difficult stools may cause hemorrhoids. Mild exercise, such as walking (inside the house or outside), often helps to get the bowel moving and will help eliminate painful gas.

### Hemorrhoids

Grape-like lumps around the rectal opening are hemorrhoids. They are often painful and itchy. During a difficult bowel movement, they may ooze bright red blood. To help bring down the swelling, try freezing a dampened maxi-pad and then putting it in your underwear. Choose to lie down, rather than sit, to take the pressure off your bottom until the hemorrhoids heal. Some of the special creams, sprays, and ointments sold to help shrink the swelling of hemorrhoids are effective. Talk to your pharmacist and doctor.

**Urination**

Immediately after the birth, or for the first day or so, you may find it hard to urinate if you had a catheter, or painful if you have stitches in place or a small tear in your vagina. To help the flow of urine get started, try turning on the taps in the bathroom sink so you can hear the water. To help take away the sting, try urinating while taking a shower or bath or squeezing warm water from a bottle over the area when you void.

Later, you may find you have to urinate quite often or that you have trouble knowing when the urine is going to start to flow. You may lose urine with a cough, sneeze, or physical activity. This problem is called urinary incontinence. It is caused by the stretching of the pelvic floor muscles. You can help strengthen your muscles by doing Kegel exercises (page 46). For most women, this problem gradually goes away.

## The shape you're in

If your abdomen is flabby and you think you still look pregnant after the birth, you are perfectly normal. Try not to worry about it. Your abdominal muscles stretched a great deal during your pregnancy and they don't just spring back into place once the baby is born. These muscles take time to slowly tighten back into their pre-pregnant shape. During pregnancy, you gained weight gradually and it may take a few months to lose it. Don't try to lose weight quickly by following a low-calorie diet. It is far better to eat a variety of healthy foods and resume exercise activity as soon as you can.

Invest in as good a stroller or carriage as you can afford (second-hand is fine), or you may be able to borrow. Look for one that is easy to walk with. Walking at a good pace is an excellent toning exercise, and your little one will enjoy it too. The latest weight-loss research has shown that as little as 20 minutes a day of brisk walking or similar exercise will affect your metabolism, so that you "burn" more calories. Severely restricting your diet will have the opposite effect, as your body adjusts to "famine conditions" by storing as much energy as possible as fat.

In some communities, you may be able to find postnatal fitness classes specifically geared to the fat-burning and toning exercises needed by new mothers. Joining these classes will allow you to meet other new mothers and talk about the things that are on your mind. If you are short of sleep and find meeting all of your baby's needs stressful, talking to other mothers about their experiences and sharing your tips and strategies will help.

Breastfeeding your baby will help you lose weight because your body needs to burn extra calories to produce the energy needed to make breast milk.

## Menstrual periods

If you are not breastfeeding, your menstrual period will start again 4–9 weeks after the birth. Your period may be longer, shorter, heavier, or lighter than before pregnancy. It should return to what is normal for you after a few cycles. If you are breastfeeding, menstruation may not start again for months or until you stop breastfeeding altogether. However, your ovaries may begin to work before your period returns. This means you could become pregnant again without ever having your period. If you wish to avoid pregnancy, you should begin using birth control as soon as you plan to resume sexual relations (usually 4–8 weeks) after the birth.

## Birth control choices

If you do not want to get pregnant, you and your partner should decide what type of birth control is best for you now. You can get pregnant while you are breastfeeding, and you can get pregnant even if your periods haven't started yet. For this reason, you should decide which birth control method is right for you and your partner, and have it ready before you begin having sex again. Talk to your doctor.

**Breastfeeding:** You can become pregnant while breastfeeding, so it is important to think about the right form of birth control for you. Breastfeeding itself will reduce your chances of pregnancy for the first six months post-partum, especially if:

• you are nursing frequently (at least every four hours);
• you do not supplement with formula;
• you have not resumed your periods.

As your baby grows older and starts on other foods, nursing becomes less frequent and your chances of getting pregnant are greater.

**Birth control pills** are a highly effective form of contraception, which you may find are a good choice after childbirth. Breastfeeding moms should use a progestin-only type of pill, as this type will have less effect on reducing milk production.  It is best not to start the pill until your breastfeeding is well established and you are producing plenty of milk.  If you are not breastfeeding, birth control pills can be started three to four weeks after delivery.

When you do start taking the pill, follow the instructions carefully. They will not be fully effective until you have completed one full cycle of pills. In the meantime, use other methods.

**Latex condoms** for men are easy to use and help protect both partners against sexually transmitted infections. They are a good choice to have on hand.

**Female condoms** are now available at your local drugstore. Be sure to follow the instructions carefully.

**Spermicidal foams and creams** kill sperm. These are most reliable when used with a latex condom. Follow the directions carefully.

**Diaphragms** cover the opening to the uterus to prevent sperm from entering. If you used a diaphragm before you were pregnant, you will need to have a new one fitted, but not until eight weeks after the birth. Diaphragms are most reliable when used in combination with spermicidal foams or creams.

**Depo-Provera®** is a highly effective injection drug used to prevent pregnancy. A health care provider will give you an injection once every three months. It is safe, easy, and economical. Talk to your doctor.

**An intrauterine device (IUD)** may be a good choice for some women, and can be fitted in the doctor's office six to eight weeks after the birth, when your uterus has returned to its normal size. Talk to your doctor.

*For more information visit the award winning SOGC website on contraception at www.sexualityandu.ca*

### If you have completed your family

**Sterilization** is permanent birth control. Although there is a possibility that sterilization procedures can be reversed surgically, you and your partner should consider your decision carefully.

**Vasectomy** is a sterilization procedure for men. A urologist (a medical specialist) will perform the procedure in his or her office under local anesthetic. In a vasectomy, a tube that carries sperm from the testicles, called the vas deferens, is cut.

**Tubal ligation** is a form of sterilization for women. It is performed in a hospital, under a general anesthetic. A number of surgical options are available. The tubes may be blocked using clips, rings, or by burning them. A newer method, done under local anesthetic, uses small metal coils to block the tubes.

## My pregnancy journal
## Your follow-up visit

Your first follow-up visit is usually 6 weeks after the birth, although your baby will likely be checked 2 weeks following birth (see Chapter Eight).

_____
_____
_____
_____
_____
_____
_____
_____
_____
_____
_____
_____
_____
_____
_____
_____
_____
_____
_____
_____

RECORDING MY PROGRESS
AFTER BIRTH OR POSTPARTUM

*Date:*
_____

*Blood pressure:*
_____

*Weight:*
_____

THINGS TO DISCUSS WITH MY
HEALTH CARE PROVIDER:

• *Am I blue (see quiz on page 121 called Recognizing signs of postpartum depression)?*

• *What are my feelings about my baby?*

• *Has my flow stopped?*

• *Am I experiencing any pain?*

• *What about sex?*

• *What about contraception?*

• *How is breastfeeding going?*

*Other concerns:*

_____
_____
_____
_____
_____
_____

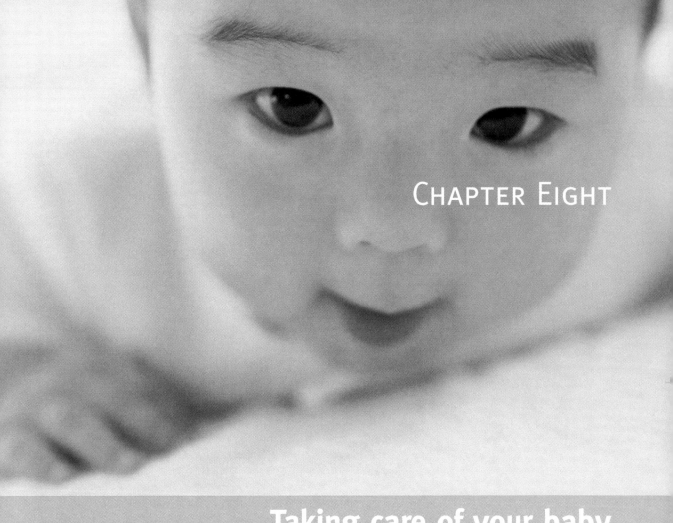

CHAPTER EIGHT

**Taking care of your baby**

## SIGNS OF DEHYDRATION IN NEWBORNS

Dehydration can be very serious. Your baby may be dehydrated if you notice any of the following signs.

▶ CALL YOUR DOCTOR IMMEDIATELY.

sunken eyes

sunken soft spot on
the top of the baby's head

drowsy, sleepy, hard to wake up

breathing faster than
40 times a minute

less urine (wets less often,
or diapers not as wet)

dark yellow urine

dry mouth, lips, tongue, nose

weight loss

fever

THIS CHAPTER WAS REVIEWED BY THE CANADIAN PAEDIATRIC SOCIETY

*Newborn babies have special needs. They need to be handled slowly, gently, and firmly. They cannot control their muscles or hold up their heads. When you pick them up you will need to support the two heaviest parts of their bodies—their heads and their bottoms. Newborn babies may have a coating of waxy vernix covering their body. When this is washed off, their skin may peel from the dryness. Many newborns have fine hair along their backs and shoulders. This usually disappears in a week or two. They may also have white spots, rashes, or blotchy skin patches that usually clear up in a few days. Some newborns have bluish-grey skin around their fingers and toes, caused by changes in their circulation after birth. Usually, this will go away in a few days.*

During the journey down the birth canal, a baby's head may be molded into an odd shape. Over the next few weeks or months, the baby's head will become a normal shape. On top of your baby's head, you will feel two soft spots where the bones of the skull have not grown together yet. These spots are called fontanelles. If you watch closely, you will see them pulse up and down. This is normal. Touching the fontanelles will not harm the baby. The bones in the skull usually grow together by the time a baby reaches 18 months of age. Some newborns have a full head of hair while others have none. Some babies may lose their hair, only to have it grow back a different colour. The colour of the baby's eyes may also change over the next three to six months.

The hormones in your body at the time of the birth may cause changes in your baby's body. For example, newborns of both sexes may develop swollen breasts when they are a few days old, and some babies' breasts leak a few drops of milk. Don't worry about this milk; it will go away by itself. Pregnancy hormones may also cause the baby's sex organs to be larger than normal for a few days. A baby boy may have a reddened scrotum (sac that holds his testicles), and baby girls may have a bit of bleeding or white discharge from their vaginas. All of these changes are normal.

## Newborn care

### Your baby's elimination

It is vitally important that your baby's elimination system is working properly. You can tell if all is well by the number of times your baby soils or wets his diaper. Newborns can become dehydrated very quickly, and this can lead to serious problems for babies. Therefore, it's very important to give your baby plenty of milk, and to make sure your baby has normal amounts of feces and urine.

Your baby's first bowel movement will be a tarry, greenish-black substance called meconium. Babies will pass meconium for about 24–48 hours after birth. After that, your baby's stool will become looser and greenish-yellow for 3-4 days.  This is called transitional stool. A breastfed baby's stool is golden yellow (like mustard). Sometimes, it will be loose or even watery, and at other times seedy, mushy, curdly, or the consistency of mustard.

Breastfed babies are rarely constipated, and may soil their diapers many times during a 24-hour period. However, some breastfed babies have bowel movements only once every few days. Formula-fed babies' feces are more solid, yellow to green in colour, and have a strong odour. Formula-fed babies tend to have more problems with constipation.

If your baby's urine is almost clear and hard to see in the diaper (but you can still feel the diaper is wet or heavier than a dry diaper), this is a good sign that your baby is getting enough milk. Very yellow urine may mean your baby is dehydrated and needs more milk (fluids). Make sure you check the diaper every time you change your baby to make sure it is wet. If there is plenty of fluid going in, then plenty of fluid (urine) should be coming out.

Newborns who lose more than seven percent of their total body fluids can become seriously ill. Read the signs of dehydration in newborns. Call your doctor if you have any concerns.

### Diapering your baby

Since newborns wet up to 18 times a day, and move their bowels as often as 10 times a day, you will need to have plenty of clean diapers on hand.

---

### SAFETY TIPS FOR CHANGING DIAPERS

1. Get everything you need before you lay the baby down to be changed.

YOU WILL NEED:

- small washcloths or disposable baby wipes;
- clean diaper and maybe clean clothes;
- ointment to prevent diaper rash.

2. Never turn your back on your baby, not even for a second!

3. Put your hand on the baby's tummy if you must reach for something. If you can't reach what you need, take the baby with you.

4. Ignore a ringing doorbell or phone, or take the baby with you to answer them.

5. Wash your hands after each time you change your baby, to prevent the spread of germs.

6. Keep a clean surface for you to change your baby on.

- *has a temperature of more than 38.5 °C (101.3 °F).*

- *has a seizure (shaking body, arms, and legs).*

- *has trouble breathing (works hard to suck air in, lips and ear lobes blue/grey coloured).*

- *has pale skin that feels cold and moist.*

- *vomits more than twice in one day (large amounts of vomit, not the spit-up kind).*

- *has diarrhea more than twice in one day (large watery stools).*

- *passes blood or blood clots.*

- *wets fewer than six diapers a day.*

- *nurses poorly or refuses to eat.*

- *seems weak, can barely cry.*

- *cries more than usual, cries differently, acts very fussy, and nothing you seem to do works to make the baby stop crying.*

- *doesn't act like he or she used to, seems "different" somehow, wakes up less alert, sleeps more than the usual amount.*

*A healthy baby can become sick very quickly. If you are concerned about your baby for any reason, call your doctor.*

To keep your baby's skin clean and dry, change your baby each time the diaper is dirty. Most parents tend to establish a diaper-changing routine. For example, some parents change the baby after each feeding, before laying the baby down for a nap. Others find that changing their baby's diaper is an effective way to wake a sleepy baby that still needs to nurse from the other breast.

There are two kinds of diapers: cloth or disposable. If you are concerned about contributing to environmental waste or the cost of disposables, then cloth diapers may be a better choice for you. Many communities have diaper services that will pick up soiled and wet diapers and deliver freshly laundered ones. If you have a washer and dryer at home, you may find washing your own is not too difficult or time consuming.

**Cord care**
The stump of the umbilical cord usually shrivels up and falls off in a week or two. The spot underneath will be the baby's belly button. Do not use any solutions when cleaning your baby's cord stump.

To keep the cord dry, fold the top of the diaper away from the stump. If the area around the cord becomes red, swollen, smells bad, or has pus coming out, the cord may be infected. Call your doctor if you think your baby's cord is infected.

**Eye care**
After the baby was born, the nurse placed special drops (or an ointment) in the baby's eyes to prevent infection from germs that could enter the eye during the birth. Unless signs of infection appear, such as redness or a discharge from the eye, all you need to do is wipe each closed eye with a moist cloth to keep the area clean. If you think the baby's eyes are infected, call your doctor or the public health nurse.

**Dressing**
Babies need the same layers of clothing as their parents are wearing. In the winter, they may need an undershirt, a shirt, and a sweater along with warm

coverings on their legs, socks or booties, and a snowsuit. In the summer, they may be most comfortable in only a T-shirt and diaper. In air-conditioned rooms or cars, your baby may need more clothes than you do because he is less active. Babies tend to feel cold sooner than you would.

**Bathing**

It is important to keep your baby clean. It is all right to give your baby a bath even if the cord has not yet fallen off. You may use mild baby soaps to clean the skin. Use a moisturizing cream to soothe dry skin. Pay special attention to the scalp and the folds in the baby's skin. For safety reasons, it is best to use a baby bathtub, not your regular tub. Gather everything you need first, and then fill the basin with about two inches of warm water. Test the water using the inside of your wrist to make sure it is not too hot, and never leave a baby alone in a tub, even for one second.

## ABOUT JAUNDICE

When some babies are a few days old, their skin and the whites of their eyes may turn a yellowish colour. This is called jaundice. Jaundice is caused by the build-up of a green substance in the baby's blood called bilirubin. Bilirubin is formed when the baby's body breaks down old red blood cells. It is the liver's job to remove bilirubin, but a newborn's liver doesn't start removing bilirubin until the baby is a few days old. During pregnancy, the mother's liver and the placenta removed the bilirubin.

If your baby becomes jaundiced you should not worry. The levels that most babies develop usually do not cause problems. High levels of bilirubin in the blood can harm a baby's nervous system, but this is rare. A baby's blood can be tested by the nurse during her home visit or by your doctor. Rarely, your baby will be treated in the hospital using phototherapy. Phototherapy is done by placing a baby under special lights. If you are discharged from a hospital within 24-36 hours of birth, the baby should be checked by a health care provider on day two or three for jaundice. In many centres in Canada, this is done by a nurse on an early home visit. If this service is not available, arrangements should be made to have your baby checked by a health professional in a clinic setting.

If you think your baby has jaundice: Feed the baby every 2–3 hours during the day and night. Call your doctor.

YOUR DOCTOR WILL WANT TO KNOW:

• the number of soiled and wet diapers your baby has had
• the quantity and colour of the stools in soiled diapers

Instructions from your doctor or health nurse:

REDUCING THE RISK OF SUDDEN
INFANT DEATH SYNDROME (SIDS)

- *For sleep, normal, healthy infants should be placed on their back.*

- *All infants should be cared for in a smoke- and drug-free environment.*

- *Infants should be dressed and covered in a manner to avoid overheating, even during an illness.*

- *Breastfeeding is the best way to feed your baby and may give some protection against SIDS.*

- *Firm flat bedding should be used for normal healthy infants, with sheets and light blankets as needed, but without products to maintain the sleeping position.*

- *Never put your baby on a water bed.*

- *Never use a comforter or a duvet in an infant's crib.*

**Sleeping – creating a safer environment**

Sudden infant death syndrome (SIDS) is the unexpected death of a baby under one year of age and occurs while the baby is sleeping. While the cause is unknown, studies have shown that there are things you can do to make the baby safer.

- Your newborn should be put to sleep on his back on a firm, flat surface. When your baby is old enough to turn over onto his tummy on his own, then it is not necessary to force him back to sleep on his back.

- The crib should be free of fluffy pillows, comforters, stuffed toys or bumper pads, which could cover the baby's face. Use lightweight blankets to keep the baby warm but not hot.

- The risk of SIDS is increased if parents smoke or if there has been consumption of alcohol or drugs while sleeping with the baby.

- Breastfeeding is associated with a lower incidence of SIDS.

(Adapted from the Canadian Paediatric Society Position Statement: Recommendations for Safe Sleeping Environments for Infants and Children (2004) and parent handout, Back to Sleep: Reducing the Risk of SIDS.)

## Circumcision

Circumcision is a surgical procedure in which skin covering the end of the penis is removed. An infant must be stable and healthy to be circumcised. The decision to circumcise may be based on personal, religious and cultural factors. After reviewing the medical evidence, the Canadian Paediatric Society does not support circumcision as a routine procedure for newborns. Since circumcision is not essential for health, parents should make a decision based on the benefits and risks.

If you choose not to circumcise, the uncircumcised penis is easy to keep clean. An infant needs only gentle washing of the genital area while bathing. The foreskin does not fully retract for several years and should never be forced. Later, when the foreskin fully retracts, boys should be taught to gently wash underneath the foreskin.

When circumcision is performed, appropriate attention needs to be paid to pain relief. After circumcision, you should contact your health care provider if your baby does not urinate within 6-8 hours, if there is persistent bleeding, or if there is redness around the tip of the penis that gets worse after three days. Further information on circumcision can be obtained from the Canadian Paediatric Society (www.cps.ca).

## Car seats

Always use a car safety seat starting from your baby's first ride home from the hospital.

All infant and child car seats sold in Canada must meet Transport Canada's safety regulations. These regulations help protect children in case the vehicle suddenly stops or is involved in a collision. Carefully refer to the instructions that come with the car seat and attach the seat as recommended to the car. The Universal Anchorage System (UAS) allows the car seat to be installed with a seatbelt in the rear seat of the vehicle. Note that a forward facing seat also requires a top tether strap. You should be cautious about buying or borrowing a used car seat. Make sure it is not missing parts or instructions. You should never use a car seat that is more than 10 years old.

▷ **Infant car seat**

### CAR SEAT SHOPPING CHECKLIST*

☐ Does the car seat have a national safety mark?

☐ Is there an instruction booklet?

☐ Is the car seat appropriate for the weight and height of your child?

☐ If the car seat has an expiry date, will the time period cover your needs?

☐ Can the car seat be installed correctly in your vehicle?

☐ Are the harness and tether straps easy to adjust?

* Adopted from Transport Canada's Keep Kids Safe: Car Time 1-2-3-4 (www.tc.gc.ca/roadsafety/tp/tp13511/tips.htm)

*This symbol for UAS marks the location of the anchor bars in the vehicle and the connectors on the car seat.*

DID YOU KNOW?

*Offering a bottle to a baby while trying to establish breastfeeding can cause "nipple confusion."*

BREAST IS BEST

REMEMBER:

*The colostrum you produce in the first one or two days is the perfect mixture for your new baby. Although small in volume, it is enough.  You do not need to supplement with formula.*

## Feeding your baby

The time you spend feeding your baby is a special time for both of you. Babies thrive on feeling your warmth and love as you hold them. They also love to suck and love the feeling of being full of warm milk. Many new mothers feel a close bond forming with their babies when they feed them. To a newborn, feeding time is heavenly.

The Society of Obstetricians and Gynaecologists of Canada and the Canadian Paediatric Society recommend breast milk as the best and only food for babies for the first six months. At six months, introduction of nutritious complementary foods is recommended while breast milk is continued for the first two years of life, or longer. No commercial formula contains antibodies, growth factors, enzymes and other components positively affecting short- and long-term health.  As for the nutritional value of formula, various important differences remain. However, babies will grow and develop well on formula too.

## Breastfeeding

Breast milk, including the colostrum of the first few days, is perfectly suited to meet the needs of your baby. It has all the right ingredients, in just the right amounts, to help her growth. It is the perfect temperature, inexpensive and always available. In addition, breastfeeding helps you to lose weight, and stimulates your uterus to shrink back to normal size. Breastfeeding helps you feel close to your baby.

At first, your breasts produce colostrum. This is a yellowish sticky milk-like substance. It is rich with vitamins, protein, and antibodies to protect your baby from infections. Newborns have a store of fat and water that they use up in the first few days of life. This explains why newborns lose weight at first. Colostrum alone is enough food for your baby for the first few days. There is no need to give your baby water or formula. Abundant milk will come in within 2-3 days.

Eating balanced meals and taking lots of fluids is important while breastfeeding. Do not diet. You will slowly lose weight. Remember that it took you nine months to gain and it will take nine months to lose and return to your pre-pregnancy weight.

**When to start**
The best time to start breastfeeding is within the first 30 to 60 minutes after the birth when your newborn is very alert and ready to suck. Your nurse will ask if you want to breastfeed your baby, and will help you get started. Not all babies learn immediately how to nurse, but it is still a good idea to use this time to get breastfeeding started. Make sure you let the hospital staff know that you want your baby to stay in your room with you (rooming in) so you can nurse your baby whenever he seems hungry. Feeding your baby frequently helps to increase your milk supply.

Your baby will gradually increase the length of time at the breast for one feeding but will demand less frequent feedings. After one or two weeks it is common for the baby to nurse on both breasts at each feeding.

## Nursing positions

You can nurse your baby in many comfortable positions. Here are a few ideas:

**Lying down**
Lie in bed on your side, with your head on a couple of pillows. Lay the baby down beside your lower breast. Put a rolled up blanket or towel behind the baby's back.

**Cradle hold**
Find a comfortable sitting position. Prop a pillow under the arm that holds your baby. Put the baby's head at your breast with the baby's feet lying across your abdomen.

LYING DOWN

CRADLE HOLD

FOOTBALL HOLD

(continued on sidebar page 141)

## BREASTFEEDING TIPS

- *Ask the nurses to make sure your baby is latching on properly before you go home.*
- *Be sure to drink water often during the day.*
- *Get comfortable before you begin nursing. Gather everything you need beforehand, so you won't have to keep getting up.*
- *Keep your baby skin-to-skin in the early days to stimulate the breastfeeding process.*
- *Keep your baby close by so you can pick up your baby's early feeding cues.*
- *Burp your baby after each feeding.*
- *Start with one breast, letting the baby nurse for as long as he likes.*
- *The baby will fall asleep, stop sucking or let go of your breast when finished.*
- *If your baby falls asleep too quickly on your breast, try using breast compression to stimulate her to drink more.*
- *Make sure that your baby is not too hot from overdressing while breastfeeding.*

### Football hold
Find a comfortable sitting position. Tuck the baby's legs under your arm so the feet point toward your back. Use a pillow to support the baby's head at the level of your breast. (This position puts less pressure on your abdomen if you had a caesarean birth.)

### How to get started
It usually takes a bit of time for both you and your baby to learn how to breastfeed. Babies naturally want to suck. When you brush your finger across the baby's cheek, he will naturally turn his head toward you and open his mouth. When you put your nipple in the baby's mouth, the baby will start to suck. This causes milk to flow. For the first 24 hours, your baby will probably nurse about every 2–3 hours for three to five minutes on each breast. Or your baby may only nurse from one breast and stop.

FOLLOW THESE STEPS TO HELP YOU GET STARTED:

### Step 1. Get comfortable.
Have pillows handy to support your arm, hold the baby close in the crook of your arm and point his face toward your breast; put your baby's abdomen against yours. Bring the baby towards you. Do not go towards the baby. You will have back pain and improper latch.

### Step 2. "Latching on."
Achieving a good "latch" is the most important step in guaranteeing successful breastfeeding without discomfort. Here are some pointers to help you:

- Roll the baby's body towards you and wait until the baby's mouth is open.
- Point the nipple towards the baby's nose. When drawing the baby towards the breast, support his/her neck and shoulders. Do not push on the baby's head. Once latched, the nose does not usually touch the breast, only the chin does.
- Put the baby onto the breast with the lower jaw well down on the areola (the dark area around the nipple) and place lots of your nipple back into the baby's mouth.

- In this way, the baby should not be sucking from the nipple but applying pressure with her jaws and tongue further back expressing milk from the storage spaces around the nipple into her mouth. You will be able to see her swallowing the milk.

◑ **A good "latch"**

**Step 3. Breaking the suction.**
To take the baby off your breast, slide your smallest finger inside the corner of the baby's mouth and push down a bit. This will break the suction seal. Do this every time you want to take the baby off your breast to prevent your nipples from becoming sore, then go back to Step 2 and try to get the baby to latch on again.

## Common breastfeeding problems

### Tender, sore breasts
Wear a properly fitting, full-support nursing bra all the time, even at night. Change nursing positions to better drain milk from all parts of your breasts. Make sure both breasts get an even amount of nursing time. The best way to care for your breasts is to make sure your baby latches on properly, every time.

### Sore nipples
During the first couple of weeks of nursing, it is normal for your nipples to feel tender when your baby first latches on to the breast. This tenderness is most noticeable as the baby latches on, decreasing by the count of ten.

*(Breastfeeding tips continued)*

- *Take a break. Burp your baby. Change a soiled diaper and wash your hands. (This often stimulates the baby to wake up and continue feeding. Nursing is tiring work for a newborn.)*

- *Start again with the other breast. If the baby won't take any more, try to remember to start with this breast next time.*

- *To help you remember which breast to begin with next feeding time, put a safety pin on that side of your bra or move a ring to that hand.*

- *You can feed your baby from both breasts each time, or you can feed your baby from one breast one time and the other breast the next time. Either way is perfectly fine. You will produce the most milk if your breasts are emptied during a feed.*

- *Feed your baby often at first to help your milk come in and prevent becoming engorged (see page 142).*

- *Babies have growth spurts around 3, 6, and 12 weeks. They will ask to be fed almost constantly for 24 to 48 hours. This is nature's way of increasing milk production.*

- *Until breastfeeding is established avoid using a bottle or soother. The two different sucking techniques confuse a baby.*

- *Taking care of a newborn is tiring work. If possible, ask for help with the baby, housework or other children.*

Once the baby is properly latched, there should be no pain. If nipple pain increases or continues throughout the entire feeding or after the feeding, this is a warning that something is wrong.

Check with the nurses on the unit or your public health nurse to be sure your technique is good. Make sure the baby latches on properly. If she has not, break the seal and get the baby to latch on again. Begin nursing on the breast that feels the least sore. Nurse often, offering the breast as soon as the baby first seems interested. Crying is a late hunger cue—but by then she may be too frantically hungry to get a good latch.

To help heal the nipple, spread a few drops of breast milk over it and let them dry in the air after each feed. Breast milk contains fat with antibacterial and antiviral properties and other substances that help heal and protect. Modified lanolin cream such as Pure-Lan® or Lansinoh® may also prove helpful. Avoid the use of soaps, which dry out the skin and wash away the skin's natural oils. Use cloth or paper breast pads in your bra to help absorb the leaking milk, but change them often so that they don't keep your nipples damp. Use a cold, wet towel or ice on your nipples between feeds to reduce swelling.

### Engorgement
Breastfeeding is a matter of supply and demand. Breasts become engorged (very full of milk) when the supply is greater than the demands of the baby. After a while, your breasts learn how much milk is needed to satisfy your baby and will not produce extra. For this reason, it is important to feed your baby regularly and not to miss any feedings. Engorged breasts may be hard, lumpy, and painful because the swollen milk glands are very full of milk. They can be so swollen that the nipple becomes flat and hard for the baby to latch on to. In this case, you will need to express some milk to take the pressure off the breast and allow the flattened nipple room to stand up.

To decrease engorgement, use cold compresses between feedings. Just before feeding, use of hot compresses can help improve milk flow. Wearing green cabbage leaves in the bra can also reduce swelling.

**Blocked milk ducts**

You may have a blocked milk duct if you notice one area of a breast that seems particularly tender, warm, and swollen. In this case, it is best to try to open the milk gland before nursing your baby, by putting warm wet towels on your breasts. Then massage your breasts in an effort to move the milk toward your nipples as you nurse your baby. Start under your arms. Make sure the baby latches on properly. Nurse your baby as often as possible to help keep the milk flowing. Increase the amount of fluids you are drinking to help flush out the milk ducts. Take Tylenol® about 20 minutes before you begin nursing. After the feeding, put cold wet towels on your breasts to reduce swelling.

**Mastitis**

Mastitis is an infection of one or more milk glands in the breast. You may experience flu-like symptoms, fever and chills, and notice a reddened, hot spot on one or both breasts. Call your doctor right away. Mastitis is a serious infection that can be easily treated with antibiotics. Get plenty of rest. It is important to continue to empty milk from a breast with mastitis. Take pain relief and continue to breastfeed as usual. If it is too painful to feed your baby from the affected breast, you should try to empty your breast regularly with gentle hand expression or a breast pump. It is not harmful to the baby to be fed from a breast with mastitis.

## What if I cannot breastfeed?

For some mothers, breastfeeding is not an option. One example is a mother who is HIV positive. Breastfeeding is not recommended as the virus may be transmitted through the mother's breast milk to the baby. Sometimes your health care provider may suggest formula feedings for medical reasons. In these cases, commercial brand-name formulas do provide your baby with the necessary calories and nutrients.

*Watch for signs of hunger
(making sucking noises, turning
head toward breast with open
mouth) and feed a hungry baby
before she starts to cry.*

*Pick up, rock, cuddle, hold, burp,
and walk a fussy baby.*

*Massage her body, sing, coo, and
talk to a lonely baby.*

*Check for a dirty diaper and change
an uncomfortable baby.*

*Take layers of clothing off a warm
baby (you can tell by feeling the
temperature of the skin on a baby's
tummy) and add layers of clothing
to a cool baby.*

*Wrap a receiving blanket
snugly around the over-tired
baby to help her sleep.*

**Choosing the right formula**

It is important to choose a commercially prepared brand name formula. If you are not sure which type to use, ask your doctor or public health nurse. Most of these formulas are made from cow's milk that has been changed to make them more digestible for babies. Some babies have trouble digesting cows'-milk-based formulas. For these babies, soy-based formulas are a good substitute. Choose a formula that is recommended for newborns, and not a formula for older babies. Formula comes in three forms: as a powder you mix with water, as a concentrated liquid you mix equally with water, and in a ready-to-serve form. Each of these forms gives your baby the same nourishment, if you mix them according to the instructions.

**Sterilizing equipment**

It is not always necessary to sterilize the equipment you will use to bottle-feed your baby, but it is very important to keep the equipment clean. Wash it well in hot, soapy water and rinse all the soap off. Leave it to air dry. Some mothers prefer to sterilize equipment until their babies are a few months old, or when their babies are sick. It is easy to sterilize the equipment. All you have to do is submerge all the equipment in a deep pot of water. Bring the water to a boil for five minutes. Remove the cooled equipment from the water with sterilized tongs (lifters) and fill it with formula.

## Why babies cry

Newborns cry a lot until they are about two months old. Crying is the only real way that very young babies have to communicate their needs and feelings (hungry, wet, tired, lonely, uncomfortable, too warm, too cold, or frustrated in any other way).

Sometimes newborn crying seems entirely unrelated to basic need. Four out of five babies have daily crying sessions lasting from 15 minutes to an hour that are not easily explained. It can be very upsetting when you can't seem to find out what your baby needs.

Sometimes, you will offer a feeding, a dry diaper, a cuddle, and everything else you can possibly think of, and she will still not stop crying. You may feel useless, frustrated, and even angry.

## What about pacifiers (soothers)?

Pacifiers have been used by many families throughout history for help in soothing their babies. Scientific studies have shown pacifier use has been associated with disadvantages such as dental problems, ear infections and early weaning from breastfeeding. On the other hand, they have proven ability to provide comfort to babies during painful procedures and have been associated with a lower incidence of SIDS. If a pacifier is used, the following advice should be considered:

- Avoid using a pacifier until breastfeeding is fully established.
- Never use a pacifier in place of feeding, comforting or cuddling the baby.
- Make sure the pacifier is clean and not damaged.
- Never dip the pacifier in sugar or honey.
- Never tie a pacifier around your baby's neck.

(Adopted from the Canadian Paediatric Society: Pacifiers (soothers): A User's Guide for Parents. Further information can be obtained from the Canadian Paediatric Society website for parents: www.caringforkids.cps.ca)

## Getting your baby immunized

Vaccines have been developed so that your baby and child need not suffer from diseases, which in the past have been (and still can be) the cause of serious illness, permanent suffering or death. Vaccines that are offered to your baby through the public health system are very safe and effective. The following is a schedule of immunizations that will be offered to your child.

**Routine immunization programs for infants and children in Canada, June 2005\***

| Province or territory | DaPT/IPV/Hib (2, 4, 6, 18 mo) | Hepatitis B | MMR (2 doses) | DaPT/IPV (4-6 yrs) |
|---|---|---|---|---|
| British Columbia | √ | 2, 4, 6 mo | 12, 18 mo | √ |
| Alberta | √ | Grade 5 | 12 mo, 4-6 yrs | √ |
| Saskatchewan | √ | Grade 6 | 12, 18 mo | √ |
| Manitoba | √ | Grade 4 | 12 mo, 4-6 yrs | √ |
| Ontario | √ | Grade 7 (2 doses) | 12, 18 mo | √ |
| Quebec | √ | Grade 4 | 12, 18 mo | √ |
| New Brunswick | √ | 0, 2, 6 mo | 12, 18 mo | √ |
| Nova Scotia | √ | Grade 4 | 12 mo, 4-6 yrs | √ |
| PEI | √ | 2, 4, 15 mo | 15, 18 mo | √ |
| NL | √ | Grade 4 | 12, 18 mo | √ |
| Northwest Territories | √ | 0, 1, 6 mo | 12, 18 mo | √ |
| Yukon Territory | √ | 2, 4, 12 mo; < 19 yrs not immunized | 12, 18 mo | √ |
| Nunavut | √ | 0, 1, 9 mo | 12, 18 mo | √ |

*DaPT Diphtheria-acellular pertussis-tetanus; dTap-diphtheria acellular pertussis vaccine; Hib Haemophilus influenzae type b vaccine; IPV Inactivated polio vaccine; MMR Measles-mumps-rubella vaccine; mo Age in months; N/A Not available; NL Newfoundland and Labrador; PEI Prince Edward Island; yrs Age in years*

*\*Adopted from the Canadian Paediatric Society Position Statement: PID Note: Immunization Update 2005: Stepping Forward.*

| dTap | Varicella | Meningococcal conjugate | Pneumococcal conjugate | Influenza |
|---|---|---|---|---|
| Grade 9 | 12 mo | 2, 12 mo | 2, 4, 6, 18 mo | 6-23 mo |
| Grade 9 | 12 mo | 2, 4, 6 mo | 2, 4, 6, 18 mo | 6-23 mo |
| Grade 8 | 12 mo | 12 mo | 2, 4, 6, 18 mo | N/A |
| Grade 9 | 12 mo | Grade 4 | 2, 4, 6, 18 mo | 6-23 mo |
| 14-16 yrs | 15 mo | 12 mo or 12 yrs or 15-19 yrs and high risk | 2, 4, 6, 15 mo | ≥6 mo |
| Grade 9 | N/A | 12 mo | 2, 4, 6, 15 mo | 6-23 mo |
| Grade 9 | 12 mo | 12 mo | 2, 4, 12 mo | 6-23 mo |
| Grade 10 | 12 mo | 12 mo | 2, 4, 6, 18 mo | 6-23 mo |
| Grade 9 | 12 mo | 12 mo | 2, 4, 6, 18 mo | N/A |
| Grade 9 | 12 mo | 12 mo | 2, 4, 6, 18 mo | N/A |
| Grade 9 | 12 mo | 2, 4 mo | N/A | 6-23 mo |
| Grade 9 | N/A | 2, 6 mo | 2, 4, 6, 12-18 mo | 6-23 mo |
| Grade 9 | 12 mo | N/A | 2, 4, 6, 15 mo | ≥6 mo |

## Common questions about vaccines

**Are vaccines safe?**
**Yes.** Vaccines are among the safest tools of modern medicine. Serious side effects are rare.

**Why do we need vaccines if the diseases they prevent have disappeared?**
Most diseases are still in existence somewhere and in countries where fewer people are immunized. Outbreaks of the disease do occur.

**Why can't I take a chance that my child will not get sick?**
Unvaccinated children have a much greater chance of getting the disease than those who have received the vaccine.

**Do vaccines weaken the immune system?**
**No.** Vaccines strengthen the immune system to protect against specific diseases.

**Can natural infection be an alternative to vaccines?**
Vaccines create immunity to specific diseases without causing the suffering of the disease itself. The diseases themselves can kill or disable children so we want to prevent getting the natural disease.

### Vaccine Safety in Canada[1]
- The vaccines used in Canada are extremely effective and safe.
- Serious adverse reactions are rare. The dangers of vaccine-preventable diseases are many times greater than the risks of serious adverse reactions to the vaccine.
- Health authorities worldwide take vaccine safety very seriously. Expert committees in Canada investigate reports of serious adverse events.
- There is no evidence that vaccines cause chronic diseases, autism or sudden infant death syndrome. Alleged links - for example between hepatitis B vaccine and multiple sclerosis - have been disproved by rigorous scientific study.

1. *Canadian Immunization Guide. Sixth Edition 2002.  Population and Public Health Branch. Centre for Infectious Disease Prevention and Control.*

## Getting help when you cannot cope

It can be a very hard job to look after a baby. You may need help. It is okay to need help. Many new mothers do. To protect your baby, you must take control of the situation and get the help you need. Never shake your baby. Even treating your baby roughly, for example by throwing the baby into her crib, can cause brain damage.

**If you are very angry and very frustrated** and you cannot cope for another second with your crying and fussing baby, you are at your wits' end and worried you may be losing your mind or losing control, or think you may hurt your baby, **put your baby in a safe place!** (in the crib or on the floor if the baby cannot crawl). Leave the room, close the door, walk to another part of the house, away from the crying baby (the baby will be fine for a few minutes even if she is crying).

**Get control over your feelings...**express your feelings by letting the rage out: hit a pillow, a mattress, yell, scream, and stomp your feet. Be angry without hurting the baby! Take a deep breath, relax, count slowly to 10. Get control of yourself.

**Get help. Now. Call someone. Don't wait another minute!**
Call someone you trust or anyone who may be able to help you find the help you need:

- a friend, family member, or your partner
- the hospital where you had your baby
- the public health nurse or your doctor

**NEVER SHAKE YOUR BABY**

WALK AWAY

CALL FOR HELP

## Parenting classes

Classes to promote good parenting are available in most communities. These classes are recommended for everyone because they help to boost the confidence of new parents. Most importantly, they offer new parents a chance to share their experiences with other parents facing many of the same problems and joys. They are particularly helpful for first-time parents or very young new parents.

In these classes, you will learn basic parenting skills, such as feeding, diapering, and bathing, in addition to a variety of other topics such as child safety, sibling rivalry, and coping with frustration. If you and your partner recently arrived from another country, parenting classes may be useful in helping you to bridge the cultural differences you may face raising a child in Canada.

Most importantly, parenting classes may be very beneficial for you if, when you think back to your own childhood, you feel saddened by the way your parents raised you and you want to do a better job with your children. Now may be your chance to break the cycle and begin afresh with your own family, as you set out on the sometimes hard, always rewarding, job of raising a healthy, happy child.

First aid and infant CPR courses are also available to take as you embark on your journey as parents. Information on these courses is available from the Canadian Red Cross or your public health centre.

**Emergency and community contact numbers:**

_____

_____

_____

_____

_____

_____

_____

_____

_____

_____

_____

_____

_____

_____

_____

_____

_____

_____

_____

_____

_____

_____

_____

# Key resources and services

Most people have some questions about their pregnancy and developing baby. Here is a selection of key resources and services about health before and during pregnancy, and in the first few weeks following delivery. A range of supports is provided, including helpful websites, documents, programs and phone lines. Finding answers to your questions is important, for your health, and the health of your baby.

**Aboriginal CAPC/CPNP**
*Phone: 1-800-361-0563 or 1-807-684-1920*
*Web: www.kanen.on.ca*

**Assaulted Women's Helpline**
*Phone: 1-866-863-0511 or 1-416-863-0511*

**Association of Ontario Midwives**
*Phone: 1-866-418-3773 or 1-416-425-9974*
*Web: www.aom.on.ca*

**Association of Ontario Translators and Interpreters of Ontario**
*Phone: 1-800-234-5030 or 1-613-241-2846*

**Best Start Resource Centre**
*Phone: 1-800-397-9567 or 1-416-408-2249*
*Web: www.beststart.org*
*Alcohol: www.alcoholfreepregnancy.ca*
*Health Before Pregnancy:*
*www.healthbeforepregnancy.ca*

**Canada Prenatal Nutrition Program**
*Web: www.phac-aspc.gc.ca/dca-dea/*
*programs-mes/index_e.html*

**Canadian Cancer Society Smokers' Helpline**
*Phone: 1-877-513-5333*
*Web: www.smokershelpline.ca*

**Canadian Centre for Occupational Health and Safety**
*Phone: 1-800-668-4284 or 1-905-570-8094*
*Web: www.ccohs.ca*

**Canadian Child Care Federation**
*Web: www.cccf-fcsge.ca*

**Canadian Coalition for Immunization Awareness and Promotion**
*Web: www.immunize.cpha.ca*

**Canadian Federation for Sexual Health**
*Phone: 1-613-241-4474*
*Web: www.cfsh.ca*

**Canadian Foundation for the Study of Infant Deaths**
*Phone: 1-800-363-7437 or*
*1-416-488-3260*
*Web: www.sidscanada.org*

**Canadian Health Network**
*Web: www.canadian-health-network.ca*
*Children's Affiliate: www.canadian-health-network.ca/1children.html*

**Canadian Mental Health Association – Postpartum Depression**
*Web: www.cmha.ca/bins/content_page.asp?cid=3-86-87-88&lang=1*

**Canadian Paediatric Society – Caring for Kids**
*Web: www.caringforkids.cps.ca*

**Centre of Excellence for Early Childhood Development**
*Web: www.excellence-earlychildhood.ca*

**Child and Family Canada**
*Web: www.cfc-efc.ca*

**Children with Special Needs**
*Web: www.children.gov.on.ca/CS/en/programs/SpecialNeeds/default.htm*

**Community Action Programs for Children**
*Web: www.phac-aspc.gc.ca/dca-dea/programs-mes/index_e.html*

**Dads Can**
*Phone: 1-888-323-7226*
*Web: www.dadscan.ca*

**Diabetes**
*Web: www.diabetesontario.org*

**DisAbled Women's Network Canada**
*Web: www.dawncanada.net*

**Doulas**
*Web: www.canadiandoulas.com*

**Family Pride Canada**
*Web: http://familypride.uwo.ca*

**Family Resource Programs**
*Phone: 1-866-637-7226 or*
*1-613-237-7667*
*Web: www.frp.ca*

**Family Service Canada**
*Phone: 1-800-668-7808 or*
*1-613-722-9006*
*Web: www.familyservicecanada.org*

**Father Involvement Initiative**
Web: www.cfii.ca/fiion

**Growing Healthy Canadians - A Guide to Positive Child Development**
Web: www.growinghealthykids.com

**Healthy Babies, Healthy Children**
Web: www.children.gov.on.ca/CS/en/programs/BestStart/Healthy/default.htm

**Healthy Ontario**
Web: www.healthyontario.com

**Immunization**
**Canadian Immunization Guide. Sixth Edition. Minister of Health**
Web: www.phac-aspc.gc.ca/publicat/cig-gci/index.html

**Infant Development Program**
Web: www.children.gov.on.ca/CS/en/programs/SpecialNeeds/infDevelopment.htm

**Infant Hearing Program**
Web: www.children.gov.on.ca/CS/en/programs/BestStart/InfantHearing/default.htm

**Invest In Kids**
Web: www.investinkids.ca

**La Leche League Canada**
Phone: 1-800-665-4324
Web: www.lalecheleaguecanada.ca

**Lamaze International**
Web: www.lamaze-childbirth.com

**Maternity and Parenting Leave**
Web: www.labour.gov.on.ca/english/es/factsheets/fs_preg.html

**Ministry of Health and Long-Term Care INFOline**
Phone: 1-800-268-1154 or 1-416-314-5518
TTY: 1-800-387-5559

**Mother Goose Program**
Phone: 1-416-588-5234
Web: www.nald.ca/mothergooseprogram

**Motherisk**
Phone: 1-416-813-6780
Alcohol and Substance Use in Pregnancy: 1-877-327-4636
Nausea and Vomiting in Pregnancy: 1-800-436-8477
HIV in Pregnancy: 1-888-246-5840
Web: www.motherisk.org

**Multiple Births Canada**
Web: www.multiplebirthscanada.org

**Multiple Births Magazine**
Web: www.twinsmagazine.com

**National Clearinghouse on Family Violence**
Web: www.phac-aspc.gc.ca/ncfv-cnivf

**Nobody's Perfect Parenting Program**
Phone: 1-705-567-5926
Web: www.phac-aspc.gc.ca/dca-dea/family_famille/nobody_e.html

**Nutrition - Prenatal**
**Health Canada Guidelines on prenatal nutrition and healthy eating.**
Web: www.hc-sc.gc.ca/fn-an/nutrition/prenatal/index_e.html

**Ontario Association of Children's Rehabilitation Services**
Web: www.oacrs.com

**Ontario Association of Speech Language Pathologists and Audiologists**
Phone: 1-800-718-6752 or 1-416-920-3676
Web: www.osla.on.ca

**Ontario College of Family Physicians**
Web: www.ocfp.on.ca

**Ontario Early Years Centres**
Web: www.ontarioearlyyears.ca

**Ontario Federation of Indian Friendship Centres**
Phone: 1-416-956-7575
Web: www.ofifc.org

**Ontario Human Rights Commission - Pregnancy and Breastfeeding Rights**
Phone: 1-800-387-9080 or 1-416-326-9511
TTY: 1-416-314-6526
Web: www.ohrc.on.ca

**Ontario Ministry of Transportation – Car Seat Information**
Web: www.mto.gov.on.ca/english/safety/carseat/choose.htm

**Ontario Poison Centre**
Phone: 1-800-268-9017 or 1-416-813-5900
Web: www.sickkids.on.ca/Poison/default.asp

**Ottawa Coalition for the Prevention of Low Birth Weight**
Web: www.lbwinfo.ca

**Our Sisters' Place – Postpartum Depression**
Web: www.oursistersplace.ca

**Parent Help Line**
*Phone: 1-888-603-9100*
*Web: www.parentsinfo.sympatico.ca*

**Perinatal Bereavement Service Ontario**
*Phone: 1-888-301-7276 or*
*1-905-472-1807*
*Web: www.pbso.ca*

**Pacific Post Partum Support Society -**
**Support Groups in Ontario**
*Web: www.postpartum.org/*
*supportgroups.html*

**Pregnancy Library**
*Web: www.pregnancylibrary.com*

**Pregnets – Smoking and Pregnancy**
*Web: www.pregnets.org*

**Prenatal HIV Testing**
*Web: www.health.gov.on.ca/english/*
*public/pub/aids/prenatalhiv.html*

**Preschool Speech and Language**
**Program**
*Web: www.children.gov.on.ca/*
*CS/en/programs/BestStart/*
*PreschoolSpeechLanguage/default.htm*

**Public Health Agency of Canada**
*Healthy Pregnancy:*
*www.phac-aspc.gc.ca/hp-gs/index.html*
*Infant Care: www.phac-aspc.gc.ca/*
*dca-dea/prenatal/index_e.html*

**Public Health Units**
*Phone: 1-800-268-1154*
*Web: www.health.gov.on.ca/english/*
*public/contact/phu/phu_mn.html*

**Safe Kids Canada**
*Web: www.safekidscanada.org*

**Sexualityandu.ca**
*Web: www.sexualityandu.ca*

**Shelternet – Shelters for Abused**
**Women**
*Web: www.shelternet.ca*

**Single Parents**
*Web: www.singleparents.about.com*

**Smoking - Resources to Help You Quit**

**Physicians for a Smoke-Free Canada**
*Web: http://www.smoke-free.ca/Y2Quit*

**The Lung Association**
*Web: http://www.on.lung.ca/getontrack/*
*getontrack.html*

**Centres for Disease Control Tobacco**
**and Information Source**
*Web: http://www.cdc.gov/tobacco/quit/*
*canquit.htm*

**Health Canada's e-Quit webpage**
*Web: http://www.hc-sc.gc.ca/hecs-sesc/*
*tobacco/quitting/e-quit/index.html*

**Health Canada's inventory**
**of cessation programs**
*Web: http://www.hc-sc.gc.ca/hecs-sesc/*
*tobacco/quitting/index.html*

**Webpage dedicated to smoking**
**cessation for pregnant women**
*Web: http://www.pregnets.org/*

**Alberta Alcohol and Drug Abuse**
**Commission**
*Web: http://tobacco.aadac.com/*

**Society of Obstetricians**
**and Gynaecologists of Canada**
*Web: www.sogc.org*

**SportCARE - Exercise and Pregnancy**
**Question Hotline**
*Phone: 1-416-323-7524*
*Toll Free: 1-866-93-SPORT*

**Telehealth Ontario**
*Phone: 1-866-797-0000*
*TTY: 1-866-797-0007*
*Web: www.health.gov.on.ca/english/*
*public/program/telehealth/*
*telehealth_mn.html*

**Transport Canada – Car Seat Safety**
*Web: www.tc.gc.ca/roadsafety/*
*childsafety/menu.htm*

**Women's Health Concerns Clinic –**
**Postpartum Depression Information**
*Web: www.stjosham.on.ca/whcc/*
*perinatal.htm*

**Women's Health Matters Pregnancy**
**Health Centre**
*Web: www.womenshealthmatters.ca/*
*centres/pregnancy/index.html*

# Resources for Families – Edmonton and Area

## Capital Health

**Capital HEALTH Link**
Phone: 408-5465
Toll Free: 1 -866-408- LINK (5465)

**Healthy Beginnings Hotline**
Phone: (780) 413-7990

**Prenatal/New Moms Network**
**Registration Line**
Phone: (780) 413-7980

For health information visit:
www.capitalhealth.ca

## Public Health Centres

**Beaumont Public Health Centre**
4918 – 50 Avenue, Beaumont
Phone: 929-4822

**Bonnie Doon Public Health Centre**
8314 – 88 Avenue, Edmonton
Phone: 413-5670

**Castle Downs Health Centre**
#214, 10807 Castle Downs Road,
Edmonton
Phone: 413-5787

**Devon Health Unit**
Suite C, 101 Erie Street S., Devon
Phone: 987-8224

**Eastwood Public Health Centre**
7919 – 118 Avenue, Edmonton
Phone: 413-5645

**Evansburg Health Unit**
4930 – 50 Avenue, Evansburg
Phone: 727-2288

**Fort Saskatchewan Health Unit**
121, 10420 – 98 Avenue,
Ft. Saskatchewan
Phone: 998-3366

**Gibbons Health Unit**
5018 – 48 Street, Gibbons
Phone: 923-3700

**Leduc Public Health Centre**
4219 – 50 Street, Leduc
Phone: 980-4644

**Mill Woods Public Health Centre**
7525 – 38 Avenue, Edmonton
Phone: 413-5685

**Morinville Health Services**
10008 – 107 Street, Morinville
Phone: 939-3388

**North Central Public Health Centre**
#25, Capital Centre Mall
9228 – 144 Avenue, Edmonton
Phone: 413-5600

**Northeast Community Health Centre**
14007 – 50 Street, Edmonton
Phone: 472-5020

**St. Albert Public Health Centre**
23 Sir Winston Churchill Avenue,
Edmonton
Phone: 459-6671

**Strathcona County Health Centre**
2 Brower Drive, Sherwood Park
Phone: 467-5571

**Thorsby Public Health Centre**
4825 Hankin Street (Box 314), Thorsby
Phone: 789-4800

**Twin Brooks Public Health Centre**
201 George P. Nicholson School
1110 – 113 Street, Edmonton
Phone: 413-5630

**Westview Health Centre**
4405 South Park Drive, Stony Plain
Phone: 968-3600

**West Jasper Place Public Health Centre**
9720 – 182 Street, Edmonton
Phone: 413-5700

**Woodcroft Public Health Centre**
13221 – 115 Avenue, Edmonton
Phone: 413-5720

**Birth Control Center**
405 Capital Health Centre
North Tower 10030 107th Street,
Edmonton
Phone: 735-0010

**Community Health Services**
**Administration**
#300, 10216 – 124 Street, Edmonton
Phone: (780) 413-7900

## Product Safety

**Health Canada Product Safety**
Phone: (780) 495-2480

**Alberta Motor Association (AMA)**
Phone: (780) 430-6800

**KIDSAFE Connection**
Phone: (780) 407-7250

## Resources for Families – Edmonton and Area – continued

### Help is Just a Call Away – 24 Hour Help for Everyone

**Emergency**

Police, Fire, Ambulance ............................................................**911**

Changing Together – A Centre for Immigrant Women ............... (780) 421-0175

Distress Line ............................................................ (780) 482-4357

Sexual Assault Centre ............................................... (780) 423-4121

Family Violence Prevention Centre ........................................... (780) 423-1635

A Safe Place (Sherwood Park) .................................................... (780) 464-7233

Stop Abuse in Families (S.A.I.F.), St. Albert ............................... (780) 460-2195

**Shelters for Women**

WIN House .................................................................. (780) 479-0058

Lurana Shelter ........................................................... (780) 424-5875

A Safe Place (Sherwood Park) .................................................... (780) 464-7233

# Suggested reading

▶ *Pregnancy Childbirth and the Newborn. The Complete Guide. (2001).*
**Authors: Penny Simkin, Janet Whalley and Ann Keppler.**

This is a comprehensive book written by renowned childbirth educators. Information is detailed, clear and supported by scientific research.

▶ *Dr. Jack Newman's Guide to Breastfeeding. (2003).*
**Authors: Jack Newman and Teresa Pitman**

This book was written by Dr. Jack Newman, a pediatrician and Canadian expert on breastfeeding and a lactation consultant (Teresa Pitman). It offers extensive practical information and encouragement on breastfeeding.

▶ *The Girlfriend's Guide to Pregnancy (1995).*
**Author: Vicki Iovine**

This book was written by a mother, television producer and host. The author discusses common issues in pregnancy with humour, light heartedness and truth. It is not a medical or scientific based handbook, but fun and helpful reading all the same.

▶ *Your Child's Best Shot. (2002).*
**Author: Ronald Gold**

This revised edition was written by Dr. Ronald Gold, a leading Canadian expert on vaccination, and answers many questions parents have on vaccination. The first version of this book was published by the Canadian Paediatric Society in 1997.

▶ *Your Baby & Child. From Birth to Age Five (2003).*
**Author: Penelope Leach**

This popular child care book covers each developmental stage – newborn, settled baby, older baby, toddler, and young child — addressing everything from feeding, teeth and teething, to growing, excreting, crying, sleeping, and playing. For each stage, an additional set of topics is discussed, including muscle power, speech, child care, and appropriate toys.

# Index

## G

genetic screening, 30-32
genital herpes/warts, 20
German measles, 18, 26
gestational hypertension, 55, 67-68,
  see also high blood pressure
gravity, centre of, 44, 59
groin, pain in, 61
group B Streptococcus (GBS), 73

## H

hair, of babies, 132
headaches, 36, 55, 67
heads, of babies, 132
heart, see also under fetus
  exercise and, 43, 45
heartburn, 60
hemoglobin, 26
hemorrhage
  during labour, 54
  postpartum, 111, 114
hemorrhoids, 59, 124
hepatitis B, 27, 28
hereditary diseases, 17
high blood pressure, 93, see also
  gestational hypertension
  premature labour and, 52
HIV, see human immune deficiency
  virus
home care, 115
hormones, 2
  babies' sex organs and, 132
  depression and, 121
  ovulation and, 4
  placenta and, 3
  pregnancy, 24
  during second trimester, 50
  sex and, 42
  skin pigmentation and, 50
hospital
  length of stay in, 115-116
  preparing for, 86, 87
  what to expect, 73-75
  when to go, 95
hot tubs, 45
human chorionic gonadotrophin
  (HCG), 3

human immune deficiency virus
  (HIV), 20, 27, 29
hydrotherapy, 103
hypertension, 67-68, see also gestational
  hypertension

## I

immature body systems, 56
immunization, 146, 147, 148
implantation, 2
indigestion, 60
induction, 89, 93-94
insulin, 41, 58, see also diabetes
intrauterine devices (IUDs), 5, 128
intravenous line (IV), 77
iron
  pregnancy and, 6
  supplements, 59

## J

jaundice, 135

## K

kangaroo care, 79
Kegel exercises, 37, 46, 120, 125
kneeling, during delivery, 103

## L

La Leche League, 70
labour, see also delivery
  body positions during, 102-103
  eating and drinking during, 78
  false, 57, 88-89, 96
  early/latent stage
  first stage, 96-106
  fourth stage, 112-113
  induced, 78, 89, 93-94
  movement during, 78
  pain control during, 21
  premature, 52-55, 56-57
  real vs. false, 88-89, 96
  second stage, 106-111
  signs of, 92
  slow progress in, 98
  stages of, 96

support during, 94-95
  third stage, 111-112
labour coaches, 74, 77, 94-95, 102
  during active labour, 100
  during early labour, 99
  during third stage of labour, 111
  during transition to active labour, 101
labour support persons, 74, see also
  midwives; obstetrical nurses
lanolin cream, 142
latching on, 140, 141
LDRP (labour, delivery, recovery, and
  postpartum) units, 74
lifestyle, of mothers, 20, 21, 29
lightening, 86
linea nigra, 50
liver disease, 28
lochia, 121
lotions, 62
lovemaking, see sexual relations
lungs
  of baby, 56, 67, 87
  exercise and, 43

## M

mastitis, 143
maternal serum screening (MSS), 30
meconium, 96-97, 133
medical history, 17, 21
  fetal abnormalities and, 30
medication
  birth control pills, 127
  during labour, 77
  for nausea and vomiting, 35
  for pain relief, 105-106
  pregnancy and, 17-18
  sleeping pills, 87
menstrual cycle, 2, 4, 25, 126
metabolism, 125
  during first trimester, 36
midwives, 33, 75, 95
milk ducts, blocked, 143
milk glands, 24
milk supply, 139
minerals, 8
miscarriages, 5, 37, 50
morning sickness, 35

Motherisk, 20, 35
mucous plug, 56, 92
multiple births, 114

## N

naps, see rest
narcotics, 105
natural childbirth, 78
nausea
  postpartum, 111
  during pregnancy, 34
neural tube birth defects, 10
nipple confusion, 138
nipples, see also breastfeeding; breasts
  soreness of, 141
nurseries, rooming in vs., 75
nursing, see also breastfeeding;
  formula feeding
  positions during, 139-140
nuchal cord translucency
nutrition, 6-7
  postpartum, 120
  during pregnancy, 38
  premature labour and, 57

## O

obstetrical nurses, 75, 95
obstetricians, 33
older mothers
  gestational hypertension
  and, 67
omega-3 fatty acids, 8, 69
ovaries, 126
overdue babies, 88, 93
ovulation, 2, 4
oxygen supply, to baby, 78, 112
oxytocin, 94, 98, 103, 114, see also
  hormones

## P

pacifiers, 145
pain relief, 21, 78, 100, 105-106
pancreas, 41
pant-pant-blow breathing,
  99, 101, 107

Pap tests, 27
parenting classes, 150
pelvis, 86
  exercises for, 45, 46, 59, 125
perineum, 108, 120
phototherapy, 135
pills, see medication
placenta, 3, 87
  aging, 89
  emergence of, 111, 114
  gestational hypertension and 67
  hormones made by, 3
  during second trimester, 50
placenta previa, 54
postpartum depression, 121
  gestational hypertension and, 67
  pregnancy and, 6
pre-eclampsia, see gestational
hypertension
pregnancy, see also trimesters
  early signs of, 3
  first, 67
  hormones, 36
  tests, 3
pregnancy journal
premature births, 5, 14, 21,
  see babies: premature
prenatal classes, 21, 33, 40, 57
progesterone, 3, 36, see also hormones
protein, 6
psyllium
pushing, 79, 101, 103, 106-107

## R

radiation, working with, 14
relaxation, see also rest; sleep
  between contractions, 100, 101
  postpartum, 120
  techniques, 57
religious beliefs, 74, 80
rest
  after delivery, 115, 120
  during exercise, 44
  during first trimester, 36
  gestational hypertension and, 68
  premature labour and, 57
  stress and, 40

Rh factor, 27
rooming in, 75, 80
rubella, 18, 26

## S

saunas, 45
second trimester, 50-64
  baby's development during, 51
  discomforts of, 59-62
  mother's body during, 50-51
seizures, 68, 134
sexual history, 20
  hepatitis B and, 28
sexual relations
  anal, 29
  ovulation and, 4
  postpartum, 122-123
  during pregnancy, 42
sexually transmitted diseases (STDs),
  20, 29
shaking, of babies, 149
shave preps, 77
show, 92
sitting position, during labour, 102
skin
  of babies, 132, 134
  dryness of, 62
  pigmentation, 50, 86
  skin to skin contact, 80
sleep
  of babies, 120, 136
  postpartum, 120
  during pregnancy, 87
  stress and, 40
smoking, 14
  during pregnancy, 52, 53
  premature labour and, 53, 57
  resources and cessation programs, 154
soaps, 62, 142
solvents, working with, 14
spermicidal foams and creams, 127
squatting, during delivery, 103
steam rooms, 45
sterilization, of equipment, 144
sterilization (birth control), 128
stitches, 120, 123
street drugs, 17, 29